Clinical Sociology: Research and Practice

Series Editor:

JOHN G. BRUHN
New Mexico State University, Las Cruces, New Mexico

This series explores key research and practice in this rapidly expanding field. Topics include ethical and legal aspects; the nature of client relationships; methods of intervention and evaluation; and the role of clinical sociology in specific settings. This open-ended series appeals to students and teachers in sociology, social work, community psychology, public health, health education, and counseling.

For further volumes:
http://www.springer.com/series/5805

John G. Bruhn • Howard M. Rebach

The Sociology of Caregiving

Springer

John G. Bruhn
Department of Sociology
Northern Arizona University
Flagstaff
Arizona
USA

Howard M. Rebach
Department of Sociology
University of Maryland
Salisbury
Maryland
USA

ISSN 1566-7847
ISBN 978-94-017-8856-4 ISBN 978-94-017-8857-1 (eBook)
DOI 10.1007/978-94-017-8857-1
Springer Dordrecht Heidelberg New York London

Library of Congress Control Number: 2014936058

Printed on acid-free paper

Springer is part of Springer Science+Business Media (www.springer.com)

For caregivers past, present and future
-JGB

To Katherine, and to my students
-HMR

"The greatest discovery of the 20th Century is that our attitude of mind determines our quality of life, not circumstances."

William James

Preface

How a society cares for its sick, disabled and elderly members reflects its values. In the United States the family, through the process of socialization, continues to model caregiving roles and teach caregiving skills to its members, and instill attitudes of responsibility and obligation for the care of extended kin and non-kin. However, societal change has changed the nature of caregiving in the U.S. Changes in the demographics of the U.S. population and in medical technology, and a broader definition of the family have created a growing need for more qualified multi-skilled and specialized caregivers, especially for seniors.

Frequently caregiving needs exceed the resources of a family, requiring management skills and resources for the care recipient that must be outsourced. Since the need for one or more caregivers in a family is often unexpected and unplanned for, family resources may be limited and prevent the provision of the level and quality of care needed. The resultant social and economic inequities may negatively impact the health and well-being of the care recipient.

Caregiving and how it is provided varies by culture. Some cultures emphasize nurturing more than others. There are cultures where there are strongly held values, beliefs and traditions of nurturing that extend throughout the lifecycle, whereas in other cultures relationships are more likely to be activated by situational need, formally structured, and contracted outside of kin networks. Changes in culture and lifestyle now give Americans more choices in how they can meet the physical and emotional needs of aging family members in lieu of, or in addition to, kin networks.

Caregiving has been acknowledged as an important national topic. It must be considered in the context of the life span with needs that vary with age, developmental levels, mental health needs, and physical health demands of both caregivers and care recipients. As the nature and functions of caregiving evolve it is a critical and salient issue in the lives of individuals in all demographic, socioeconomic, and ethnic categories. The "graying" of the baby boom generation, whose members turned 50 in 1996, have created new caregiving needs. Baby boomers are projected to live longer than any previous generation and the number of people aged 65 or older is expected to double between 2000 and 2030. Elderly people will also increase as a proportion of the population, and people aged 85 years and older will be the fastest growing segment of that group. Other dynamics within the older population suggest more intensive caregiving demands as well. For example, today's increased life expectancies mean that many 65 year-olds will be caring for their 90 year-old parents.

This text frames caregiving as a sociological issue focused around a number of central concerns:

- Caregiving is a life span experience associated with aging and the roles of spouses and adult children.
- Caregiving involves a complex of social system variables that influence social support and the services offered to caregivers and care recipients.
- The nature of the relationship between family caregivers, professional caregivers, and the care recipient are embedded in their interactions and dynamics influenced by the internal and external variables that inhibit or facilitate the care situation.
- Caregiving needs to be integrated with a national public health agenda.
- We need to identify and minimize the disparities or inequalities that exist in caregiving in the United States.
- How does caregiving fit within the Patient Protection and Affordable Care Act of 2010?

This text proposes to: (1) provide an overview of the growing complex issues of caregiving in the twenty-first century in the U.S.; (2) highlight the dynamics of caregiving that characterize high quality care; and (3) discuss the development of a new national model of healthcare with respect to caregiving policies and remaining barriers to care. Written for a graduate level audience in sociology, social work, psychology, anthropology, public health, gerontology and geriatrics, and public policy, some parts of the text will also appeal to lay persons in general. Our intention was to make this text a resource of information, thought, discussion, and action.

JGB
HMR

Acknowledgments

Caregiving is a serious and growing issue as we age and experience increasing health problems which often require assistance from others in negotiating the tasks of daily living, and in some cases complete dependency requiring institutional care. When caregiving involves us personally, especially, we look to resources to assist us. It was the lack of literature in the social and behavioral sciences with respect to caregiving that motivated us to undertake this text. We received encouragement from many colleagues, professional caregivers, and community organizations and agencies to write this book. We draw upon many of their ideas, experiences, and stories. The staff at Hospice of the Valley in Phoenix and their periodic continuing education workshops for volunteers were very helpful. One of the authors (JGB) has been a respite hospice caregiver for 10 years, and facilitated a grief support group for 4 years, and served as a hospital chaplain for 9 years. Both of us have had experience caring for several aged family members. Many of the caregivers in group homes and families of clients receiving assisted services contributed to this book by sharing their journeys about caregiving with us.

We thank Tracy Grindle for her superb work as typist and editor. Vince Colburn and Bob Rebach both provided their skills as graphic artists. The staff at the Frederick Douglass Library at the University of Maryland Eastern Shore Campus were generous and helpful in providing resource material for this book.

Acknowledgments

Contents

List of Figures

List of Tables

Chapter 1
The Contemporary Challenges of Caregiving

1.1 Introduction

When physical or mental illness or the effects of aging or other forms of disability affect family members who require care, families in most cultures have traditionally provided care for their dependent members (Olson 1994). This is not new. What is new is the growing recognition among health services providers and some public policy makers in the U.S. that caregiving needs will become increasingly significant in the future because demographic, economic, and social trends of the early twenty-first century are expected to continue.

1.1.1 Trends Shaping Future Caregiving

The U.S. Government estimates suggest that the number of people using long term care services could nearly double, increasing from 15 million in 2000 to 27 million in 2050 (U.S. Department of Health and Human Services (HHS) and the U.S. Department of Labor (DOL) 2003). Estimates from national surveys concur with the number of people aged 70 and over with activity limitations and needing care expected to double from 2020 to 2050 (National Academy on an Aging Society 2000). See Fig. 1.1.

Friedland (2004) has calculated that the number of people likely to need long term care after 2015 will increase substantially faster than the numbers of people available either as family or as paid caregivers. Families will need more support to supplement their efforts and more paid caregivers will be needed to provide this support. When families are no longer able to carry the load of chronic illness and disability care, who will replace them? See Fig. 1.2.

As the demand for long–term care services is increasing in the U.S., the traditional supply of both paid and unpaid caregivers is decreasing. The majority of long-term care workers are women between the ages of 25 and 54. While the population of age 85 and older is the fastest growing age group in the U.S., the number of women aged 25 to 54 is expected to remain unchanged from 2000 to 2030

J. G. Bruhn, H. M. Rebach, *The Sociology of Caregiving*,
Clinical Sociology: Research and Practice, DOI 10.1007/978-94-017-8857-1_1,

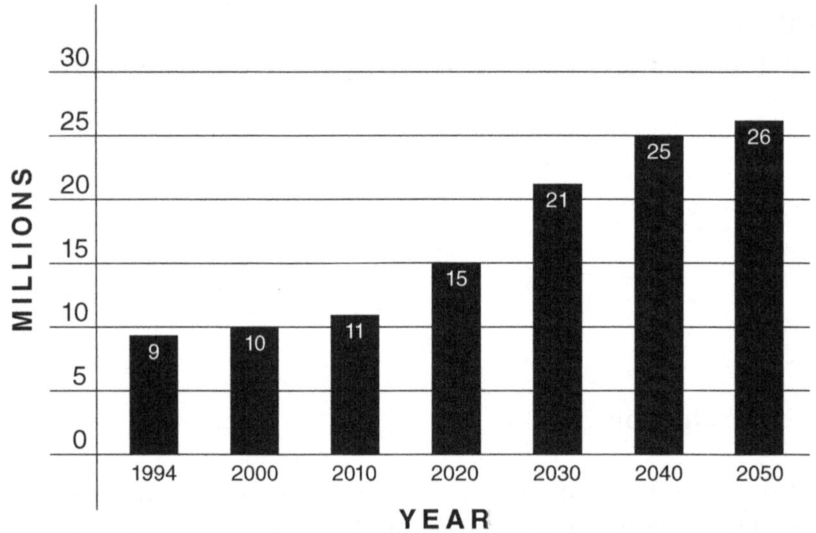

Fig. 1.1 Projected number of people age 70+ needing care. (Source: National Academy on an Aging Society analysis of data from the *1993 study of Assets and Health Dynamics Among the Oldest* Old and U.S. Census population projections (middle series))

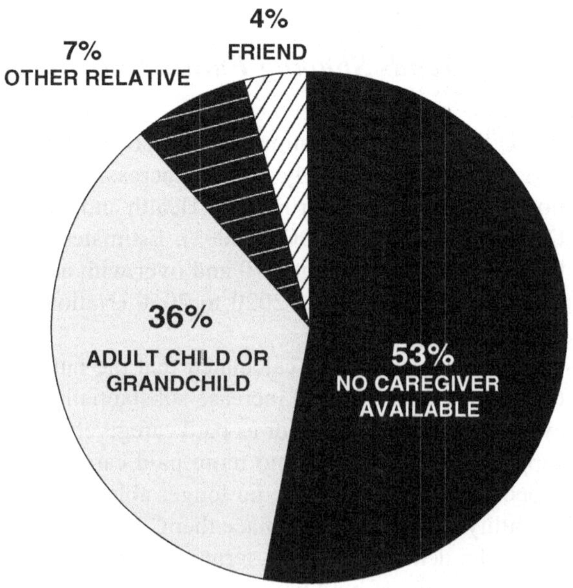

Fig. 1.2 Availability of caregivers in the future. (Source: National Academy on an Aging Society analysis of data from the *1993 study of Assets and Health Dynamics Among the Oldest Old*)

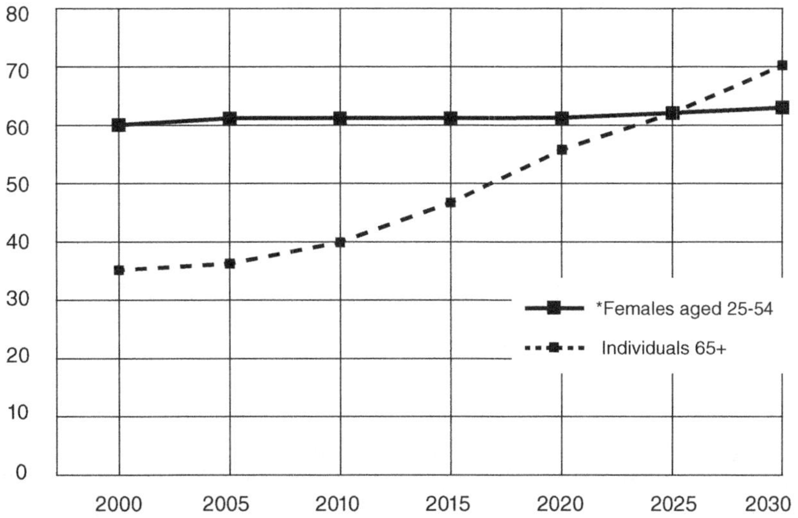

Fig. 1.3 Women of caregiving age* and individuals 65 and over in the United States, 2000–2030 (in millions). (Source: U.S. Census Bureau, National Population Projections, Summary Files, "Total population by age, sex, race and Hispanic origin")

(Fig. 1.3). Projections show a widening gap between the number of people likely to need care and the number of people who are most likely to provide care.

A number of trends are shaping the future of caregiving. Life expectancy and the aging of the U.S. population have increased dramatically during the past century. In the U.S., the equivalent of a small town of about 7,918 persons turns 60 every day (U.S. Census Bureau 2006). The global population, especially in developing countries, is aging at an even faster rate of about 795,000 persons becoming 60 years of age or older a month (Kinsella and Velkoff 2001). By 2050 the number of older persons in the world will exceed the number of youth for the first time in the history of the world.

The U.S. Census Bureau reports that the nation's population will not only be older in 2050, but will be more racially and ethnically diverse. Minorities, now representing about one third of the U.S. population, are expected to become the majority by 2042, with the nation projected to be 54 % minority by 2050. The largest growth rates are expected among Hispanics, followed by Asian–Pacific Islanders, Native Americans, and African Americans. Cultural background exerts a significant influence on caregiver's attitudes, beliefs and behaviors (Lehman 2009). See Table 1.1.

A shift in the epidemiology of disease from acute to chronic diseases has resulted in an increase in the number of persons with functional and mobility limitations who need care. The number of multigenerational families has increased, resulting in a growing number of elderly caregivers as well as an increased number of young parents who support their own children while also caring for their elderly parents, i.e.

Table 1.1 Percentage of caregivers in U.S. by gender, age and race. (Source: Caregiving in the U.S. Report by National Alliance for Caregiving and AARP, April 2004)

	Total	White	Black	Hispanic	Asian
Gender					
Male	39 %	38 %	33 %	41 %	54 %
Female	61 %	62 %	67 %	59 %	46 %
Age of caregivers					
18–34	26 %	22 %	35 %	33 %	38 %
35–49	32 %	32 %	36 %	33 %	27 %
50–64	30 %	31 %	24 %	24 %	27 %
65 and older	13 %	15 %	5 %	10 %	8 %
Mean years	46 years	48 years	41 years	43 years	42 years

the sandwich generation. Providing care for dependent family members has become increasingly difficult as greater numbers of women, the traditional caregivers, work outside the home. New forms of families, or what is known as "wider families," have changed primary relationships among family members extending formal legal rights and obligations to persons who are technically unrelated to one another (Marciano and Sussman 1991).

Social changes in the definition of what is a family also have implications for caregiving in the future. The traditional model of a married man and woman living with their own children seems to be occurring with decreasing frequency. In 1990, husband-wife households were the majority—55.2 %—which decreased to 48.4 % according to the 2010 census. Single females, no spouse present, increased from 11.6 % in 1990 to 13.1 % in 2010. Even single male heads of household, no spouse present increased from 3.4 % in 1990 to 5.0 % in 2010. Unmarried couples cohabiting increased from 5.2 % in 2000 to 6.6 % in 2010, the latter including 0.8 % of same sex couples. In 1990, 26.6 % of all births were to single women which increased to 33.2 % in 2000 and to 40.6 % in 2008 (U.S. Census Bureau 2012). It is difficult to say what these changes mean for caregiving in 2030 or 2050 but it raises questions about who will be available to provide family-based caregiving as the need for it arises for the present generations (Super 2002).

Alternatives to home-based care are often too expensive for many families with one or even two breadwinners to consider. Divorce probabilities are expected to remain at 50 %, but higher for blacks and for the less educated. Divorce puts greater distance between parents and their children and will have effects on contacts when the children become adults. Changes in healthcare reimbursement and medical technology have shifted the burden of post-acute care to family caregivers. Increased geographic mobility from rural to urban areas has distanced adult children from chronically ill siblings and/or parents (Brubaker et al. 2012).

As a result of these and other factors such as pressure from healthcare providers and the courts, dependence on family and other sources of caregiving has reached a peak (Talley and Crews 2007). For example, the U.S. Supreme Court's Olmstead decision encouraged this trend, mandating that states provide care for the elderly and individuals with disabilities in the least restrictive environment possible (Olmstead Act 1999). When caregiving is viewed as an issue that affects the quality of life for millions of individuals, it becomes both a sociological and a public health matter.

Caregiving as a growing social problem is reflected in a few of the findings from a recent national study in the U.S. funded by the MetLife Foundation and conducted for the National Alliance for Caregiving. It was reported that almost one-third of the U.S. adult population, 29 % or 65.7 million individuals, is a caregiver (National Alliance for Caregiving and AARP 2009).[1] One in seven caregivers provide care, over and above regular parenting, to a child with special needs. Seventy-eight percent of adults living in the community and in need of long-term care depend on family and friends as their only source of help. Forty-seven percent of working caregivers indicated an increase in caregiving expenses that has caused them to use all or most of their savings. Family caregivers experiencing extreme stress have been shown to age prematurely. This level of stress can shorten a caregiver's life by 10 years (Caregiving Statistics 2009).

1.1.2 Caregiving Defined

We define a caregiver as a person who provides paid or unpaid assistance and support to another person who, for reasons of illness, disability, and/or age, cannot independently perform the usual activities of daily living. At its core, caregiving is a dynamic interactive relationship between the caregiver(s) and care recipient. The caregiving role usually emerges out of an existing role relationship, usually a family role. Roles, role demands and expectations are shaped by the context established by existing social arrangements. They are further shaped by the persons' interactive history together, which often requires that role relationships be renegotiated in the context of the care situation. This could happen when a son or daughter has to exert authority toward a parent.

In addition to recognition of the presence of the relationship, caregiving should be recognized as a complex, multidimensional activity. For example, the caregiving situation can vary by the extent to which both formal and informal caregivers are involved. Formal care refers to professionals while informal care usually refers to non-professionals such as family members, friends, neighbors, and community volunteers. Thus professionals may provide health services, financial aid resources, mental health services or other community or professional resources.

A second aspect is identification of primary and non-primary caregivers where "primary" refers to the person or persons who take the major share of the responsibility and decision making as well as providing resources. This raises issues of whether care is done by a sole provider or is the caregiving shared with others such as members of a family network who provide resources of time, money and support.

[1] *Caregiving in the U.S., 2009* is based primarily on quantitative telephone screenings of 6,806 adults and interviews with 1,480 caregivers age 18 or older. Caregivers were defined as those who provide unpaid care to an adult or child.

Next, care can be provided in someone's home, or in a facility or institution, or in some combination. Formal care can be provided in the home; in-home services can include home health aides, respite care, and/or homemaker services. Care away from home can include hospice care, a group home, nursing home, or one of many forms of assisted living arrangements. Individuals can receive a mix of formal and informal and in-home and away from home services as needs change. Many facilities offer residents a venue of services that depend on their degree of dependence and mobility.

1.1.3 Changing Families and Changing Caregiving Needs

"Family" denotes a special personal relationship with the care recipient, one based on birth, adoption, marriage, or declared commitment (Levine 2004). "Caregiver" describes the job, which may include providing personal care, carrying out medical procedures, managing a household, and interacting with the healthcare and social service systems on another's behalf. However, caregivers are more than the sum of their responsibilities; they are people with complex and often conflicting felt obligations and responsibilities in the humanistic care of another person.

While family is the basic organizing structure of human societies, definitions of family have varied by culture and changed with societal characterizes and demographics. Much of what has been known as family caregiving has changed, especially since the turn of the twenty-first century. Americans aged 65 and older have tripled since 1900, from 3.1 to 35 million (U.S. Census Bureau 2001). Old age is accompanied by diseases of aging; the older one gets the greater the likelihood of acquiring more than one chronic disease. Chronic diseases have increased among Americans generally paralleling the population's lifestyle changes. Over the past five decades family caregiving has been greatly affected by the cultural, political, and economic changes in American society. "Family" today is multigenerational, biracial, nuclear, blended, gay, lesbian, and their children step and adopted, and partners. Similarly, meeting caregiving needs today usually involves multiple family helpers and a social support network. Even in cultures where the nuclear family is predominant and strong, communities have helped or assumed some caregiving roles such as helping new mothers or caring for the dying (Levine 2004). Institutions have a history of caring for individuals when family members are deceased and resources are spent. And institutions have become more specialized, appealing to persons with special needs and long term care.

Realities of twenty-first century America have profoundly changed the assumptions underlying family caregiving and earlier patterns of caregiving. The human and social costs of maintaining a family member at home now are very high. Yet, most people who need long-term care prefer to receive assistance and services at home and stay in their communities for as long as possible. Informal care is still the most important source of care for most older people.

1.1.4 Formal Caregiving

Every care recipient's situation is unique and can change according to variations in the amount of dependency experienced. In a study of 18,136 older adults, it was found that various factors influenced the utilization of formal resources, including mental status, race, age, and education (Ozawa and Tseng 1999). Younger, well-educated, single or widowed adults were more likely to utilize out-of-home services. White older adults were more likely to use in-home services compared to nonwhites. Married adults were less likely to receive formal services than non-married due to the informal supports more available to married adults. Spouses are a more likely resource than are children. Consequently, older, divorced or widowed individuals with children may use formal resources to a greater extent than older, married persons without children. Little information exists regarding the ways in which formal services are provided or how various racial and ethnic populations respond to these services and programs. However, research in this area indicates that older persons of color are less likely to use formal services than are white elderly. It has been suggested that for some individuals and families of color, feelings about formal services have been influenced by experiences of discrimination and a lack of input into the development of formal services (Toseland and McCallion 1997). For Hispanic elderly, a language barrier may deny access to programs that could be available to them (Hildreth and Williams 1996). Elderly African Americans and Hispanic families, more than white elderly, are dependent upon formal support systems and federal programs such as social security, Medicare, and Medicaid (Dilworth-Anderson and Williams 1996).

1.1.5 Informal Caregiving

Much of the care given to ill, disabled, or aging family members in the home is, for example, informal and routine personal care, and considered to be a part of their role as an able family member. Therefore, it is estimated that as many as 75 % of family caregivers who provide personal care do not self-identify themselves as caregivers until personal care and homemaker assistance becomes an economic and psychological burden. Informal care also includes transportation to healthcare appointments, shopping for groceries, paying bills, and communication within family networks.

In 2009, about 42.1 million family caregivers in the U.S. provided care to an adult with limitations in daily activities and about 61.6 million provided care at some point during the year. The estimated economic value of their unpaid contributions was approximately $ 450 billion in 2009, up from an estimated $ 375 billion in 2007. Family support is a key factor in remaining in one's home and in the community. However, if family caregivers are no longer available, the economic cost to the U.S. healthcare and long-term care services and support systems would increase astronomically (Feinberg et al. 2011).[2] The impact on the mental and emotional demands on caregivers is reflected in their health status and mortality. Caregiving stress can shorten a caregiver's life by as much as a decade, 40 to 70 % of family caregivers show clinically significant symptoms of depression, 72 % of family caregivers reported not going to the doctor as often as they should, 63 % reported poor eating habits, and 23 % of family caregivers caring for loved ones for five years or more reported their health as fair or poor (National Alliance for Caregiving and AARP 2009).

These findings provide evidence that care work has substantial effects on caregiver health. Similar results were reported by Wakabayashi and Donato (2006). They conducted an 8-year longitudinal study of women who were long-term caregivers for their parents. Their results also showed significant decline in caregiver health. This suggests a need for attention to ways that caregivers manage problematic role combinations. The health and other effects of caregiving prompted Wakabayashi and Donato to suggest:

> What is needed to enhance and support the long-term care of the elderly is a system that supports caregivers. Such a system must include the expansion of home- and community-based services, which may include the provision of meals and transportation as well as respite (day-care or home-care) services. All of these services may reduce the burden of elder care for families, allowing them to postpone or avoid the institutionalization of their elderly relatives (Wakabayashi and Donato 2006, p. 271).

1.1.6 Role Theory and Caregiving

Caregiving is a dynamic, evolving role influenced by the personal relationship between the caregiver and care recipient and their expectations, the context (formal or informal) in which care is given, the changing nature of the recipient's health, needs, and economic constraints, and family dynamics and expectations. These factors help to shape what is known as the caregiver's identity (Montgomery et al. 2007). According to caretaker identity theory, the caregiving role emerges out of an existing role relationship, usually a familial role. As needs of the care recipient change over time, care changes in quantity and intensity along with expectations from family and care recipients. Caregiving is a process linked to the progress of the care recipient's decline; it is a role requiring many different skills at different points in the care protocol of a care recipient (Pavalko and Woodbury 2000).

Montgomery et al. (2007) have identified five phases of the caregiving career that are linked to changes in the care recipient's need for assistance. Phase I of the career is the period of role onset. This period begins at the point that a caregiver assists the care recipient in a manner that is usually not a part of the caregiver's familial role. In this phase a caregiver may not be aware that they are acting as a

---

[2] For selected current national caregiver statistics and a comprehensive list of references see Family Caregiver Alliance, National Center on Caregiving, http://www.caregiver.org/caregiver/jsp/print_friendly.jsp?nodeid=439.

caregiver. Phase II is the point of self-identification as a caregiver. Phase III is when the care needs of the care recipient increase beyond the normal boundaries in the family and require a caretaker so that caretaking dominates the relationship. Phase IV can exist over an extended period of time until the care recipient's needs exceed those the family caretaker can provide. Phase V is when the care recipient is moved to a setting relieving the family caretaker of primary responsibility for caregiving.

Montgomery and his colleagues pointed out that there is often great variation in time lapse between phases of the caregiving careers and it is seldom a smooth process. The only uniform aspect of caregiving is that caregivers often experience significant distress at points of transition in their role.[3]

Usually we think of a caregiver ministering to one care recipient. However, caregivers can range from lifetime parental caregivers of adults or children with intellectual or physical disabilities who may also become caregivers to other family members (Perkins and Haley 2010), to a caregiver ministering to multiple care recipients with various conditions and needs in a group home or other institutional setting. Multiple roles provide both opportunities and consequences. Therefore, to narrow the focus of care and maximize a caregiver's knowledge and skills, some caregivers may develop specialized competencies within caregiving, such as disability care, dementia care or hospice care.

The nature of the relationship of the care recipient to the caregiver(s) can be an important dimension. Is the recipient a parent, a grandparent, sibling, spouse, child, or another relative such as an aging aunt or great aunt or is the person "fictive kin," persons not actually related but always treated as family.

1.1.7 Life Span Development and Intergenerational Caregiving

Former First Lady Rosalyn Carter (1994) said, "There are only four kinds of people in the world—those who have been caregivers, those who are currently caregivers, those who will be caregivers, and those who will need caregivers" (Carter and Golant 1994, p. 3). Almost everyone will have some encounter with caregiving in their lifetime. Individuals are increasingly assuming the role of caregiver in all phases of the life span. For example, it is estimated that there are 22.9 million caregiving households in which 8.5 million also have youth under the age of 18 living at home, many of whom assist in caregiving activity. Four million young people have developmental disabilities and another 10 million have chronic illnesses, of whom about 10 % require significant support services (LaMorey 1999). Youth who receive care are likely to have siblings who share in giving them care. Research has found that some children have begun caretaking activities for a parent before age 10 (Shifren 2008). Parentification in child caregivers can include role reversal, where the child acts as if he or she were the parent. There is concern about the impact of early

[3] Gail Sheehy, in her recent book, *Passages in caregiving: Turning chaos into confidence*, Harper Collins, 2011, emphasizes that the biggest mistake a caregiver can make is to do it alone. She says a caregiver must have a "circle of care" which consists of family, friends and professionals.

caregiving on the development of children (Shifren 2009). Longitudinal research is needed on the development of individuals who acquire the elder caregiver role early in terms of other family roles (marital, parental) and personal decisions (career, further education) (Dellmann-Jenkins and Blankemeyer 2009).

At the opposite and of the life span, over the past 30 years, the nation experienced a 118 % increase in grandparent—grandchild co-residence. In many of these families, grandparents have the sole responsibility for the grandchild (Patrick and Goedereis 2009). Several factors are responsible for the grandparents' major caregiving role, including (1) increased substance abuse in the parent generation, (2) incarceration of parents (especially mothers), (3) HIV/AIDS, (4) single parent households, (5) long work hours and job demands of the middle generation, (6) high rates of childbirth among adolescents, (7) military service, (8) and legal preference for kinship care over foster care.

For many grandparents assuming the caregiving role was a gradual process influenced by substance abuse, domestic violence, and employment situations. Grandparent caregivers often report feeling off-time from their peers who are no longer involved in daily child care as well as feeling off-time from the parents of the grandchild's classmates who are younger and engaged in normal child care. Another unique aspect of grandparent caregiving is the frustration related to different norms for child behavior and parenting across generations. The grandchildren also pose caregiving challenges. Furthermore, about half of all grandparent caregivers are raising more than one grandchild (Patrick and Goedereis 2009).

The life course stage of both caregiver and care recipient establishes another important dimension. As Aneshensel et al. (2004) noted, the idea of life course includes, "… the concept of linked or interdependent lives…" (p. 423).

> The lives of family caregivers and older care-recipients are linked long before the need for care arises, joined by bonds of marriage or by the lifelong connection between parent and child. When a spouse or parent needs care, these ordinary family roles are transformed into a specialized role characterized by new norms (Aneshensel et al. 2004, p. 423).

Therefore, variations of the care setting include older adults who care for even older frail elderly parents or grandparents, or midlife parents who care for children or adults with developmental disabilities or chronic mental illness. More generally, in the interaction between the caregiver(s) and the care recipients, it is the nature of their connection and their positions in their life courses that frame their involvement, needs, and the available resources as well as shaping the consequences for each. As Haynes (2008) wrote, caring for her mother was not an option, but a duty. Still, as research by Wakabayashi and Donato (2006) showed, women caring for elderly parents in an earlier life stage significantly increased women's risk of poverty in a later life stage.

Finally, in this brief review of the dimensions of caregiving, we must include the macro social arrangements that form the context to which all persons will have to adapt. These include various policies and legislation at local, state, and federal levels that affect the national economy and the provision of healthcare and social services as well as policies that either support or fail to support families providing care.

The case of “Kate,” age 93, illustrates this last point. Kate is an insulin-dependent diabetic, virtually blind as a result of age related macular degeneration, and immobile. Her preference was to remain in her home, and for a year her married daughter, an only child, was able to cobble together in-home services to allow Kate to remain in her home. But by the end of the year, family resources had been depleted. In addition, Kate’s health situation worsened to the point where 24 h in-home professional supervision was needed. The cost of in-home care was beyond the ability of Kate and her family members to afford. Although Kate’s only income was Social Security, ($ 1,300 per month) the state refused to provide assistance to help support her at home because, they said, her income was too high to qualify her for assistance. So, institutionalization resulted at a cost to taxpayers somewhere near twice what in-home support would have cost.

1.2 New and Continuing Challenges

Increases in life expectancy mean that more parents will survive into old age and will require care from their adult children. More adults will survive with the cumulative effects of chronic diseases, which may require specialized and full-time care from professionals in a facility. More family caregivers and care recipients will face difficult decisions about the limitations of care given family resources. More caregivers will occupy multiple roles and role conflict, role strain, role overload, and quality of care may affect decisions (Dorius and Wray-Lake 2008).

As a result of changes in family size, intergenerational relationships and caregiving will likely change: (1) these changes may lead to an earlier identification of adult caregivers; (2) an increasing number of childless individuals and couples will limit family caregivers; (3) fewer children will influence the amount and type of caregiving children can commit to; (4) family safety nets will likely be strained financially and emotionally; (5) new family forms will have an impact on intergenerational caregiving, challenging some norms of obligation and reciprocity; and (6) increased immigration will present challenges to public policy as the cost of care, cultural values, and available resources complicate choices (Wagner and Niles 2005).

1.3 Summary

As our population ages, caregiving is expected to affect all members of American society. Although family caregivers are usually untrained for the tasks they perform, they provide about 80 % of all long-term services in the U.S. Currently about 46 million Americans are providing care to an adult relative or friend. Approximately two-thirds of Americans expect to be caregivers in the future. Yet most people are not making plans for caregiving; few have purchased disability or long-term care insurance or investigated arrangements beyond the informal care provided by their immediate family. An estimated 8 million adults say they have no one to care for them.

Caregiving is a dynamic, complex role that involves continuous adaptation by caregivers and by care recipients. Caregiving can range from lifetime parental caregivers of adults and/or children with disabilities to short-term informal care of family members or friends. The type, length and intensity of caregiving can greatly influence the caregivers' identity, health, and longevity.

Individuals are increasingly assuming the role of caregiver in all phases of the life span. Children and adolescents are caring for their ill parents, parents are caring for their adult children and aging parents, and grandparents are caring for their grandchildren. Intergenerational caregiving is often accompanied by role conflict, role strain, and role overload as life span role development often lags or exceeds the expectations of caregivers seeking to bridge the gaps created by changing family dynamics and family members' perceptions of role obligations and responsibilities.

1.4 Questions for Discussion

1. How will the increasing need for future caregivers be filled? Discuss.
2. Discuss the pros and cons of rationing healthcare as one of the ways of controlling healthcare costs.
3. Discuss how caregiving needs differ among ethnic groups.
4. What national programs and policies are needed for support services in the face of the increasing costs of long term care? Discuss.
5. Have you or your family been caregivers? What were some of the issues that presented the biggest challenges for you and the care recipient?

References

Aneshensel, C. S., Botticello, A. L., & Yamamoto-Mitani, N. (2004). When caregiving ends: The course of depressive symptoms after bereavement. *Journal of Health and Social Behavior, 45,* 422–440.

Brubaker, E., Brubaker, T. H., Biegel, D. E., & Wieder, B. L. (2012). Caregiving—formal, informal. http://family.jrank.org/pages/202/caregiving.html. Accessed 10 April 2012.

Caregiving Statistics (2009). http://www.nfcacares.org/who_are_family_caregivers/care_giving_statistics.cfm. Accessed 10 April 2012.

Carter, R., Golant, S K. (1994). *Helping yourself help others*. New York: Three Rivers Press.

Dellmann-Jenkins, M., & Blankemeyer, M. (2009). Emerging and young adulthood and caregiving. In K. Shifren (Ed.), *How caregiving affects development: Psychological implications for child, adolescent, and adult caregivers* (pp. 93–117). Washington, DC: American Psychological Association.

Dillworth-Anderson, P., & Williams, S. W. (1996). African American elderly. In T. H. Brubaker (Ed.), *Vision 2010: Families & aging* (vol. 4, 1st ed., pp. 32–33). Minneapolis: National Council on Family Relations.

Dorius, C. R., & Wray-Lake, L. (2008). Expanding the horizon: New directions for the study of intergenerational care and exchange. In A. Booth, A. C. Crouter, S. M. Bianchi & J. A. Seltzer (Eds.), *Intergenerational caregiving* (pp. 351–381). Washington, DC: The Urban Institute Press.

Feinberg, L. F., Reinhard, S. C., Houser, A., & Choula, R. (2011). *Valuing the invaluable: 2011 update the growing contributions and costs of family caregiving*. Washington, DC: AARP Public Policy Institute.

Friedland, R. B. (2004). Caregivers and long-term care needs in the 21st century: Will public policy meet the challenge? Issue brief. Georgetown University Long-term care financing project July, 2004. ltc.georgetown.edu. Accessed 11 April 2012.

Haynes, Y. (2008). Not an option but a duty: Caring for my mother. In J. O. Beckett (Ed.), *Lifting our voices*. New York: Columbia University Press.

Hildreth, G. J., & Williams, N. (1996). Older Hispanic families. In T. H. Brubaker (Ed.), *Vision 2010: Families & aging* (vol. 4, 1st ed., pp. 34–35). Minneapolis: National Council on Family Relations.

Kinsella, K., & Velkoff, V. A. (2001). *An aging world. (U.S. Census Bureau, Series P95/01-1)*. Washington, DC: U.S. Government Printing Office.

Lamorey, S. (1999). *Parentification of siblings of children with disability of chronic disease: Burdened children*. Thousand Oaks: Sage.

Lehman, D. (2009). 21st century caregivers: Diversity in culture. *Aging Well, 2*(March–April), p. 26. http://www.agingwellmag.com/archive/030209p26.shtml.

Levine, C. (Ed.) (2004). *Always on call: When illness turns families into caregivers*. Nashville: Vanderbilt University Press.

Marciano, T. O., & Sussman, M. B. (Eds.). (1991). *Wider families: New traditional family forms*. New York: Haworth Press.

Montgomery, R. J. V., Rowe, J. M., & Kosloski, K. (2007). Family caregiving. In J. A. Blackburn & C. N. Dulmers (Eds.), *Handbook of gerontology: Evidence-based approaches to theory, practice, and policy* (pp. 426–454). New York: Wiley.

National Academy on an Aging Society (2000). *Caregiving*, No. 7, May, 2000. Washington, DC. http://www.agingsociety.org/agingsociety/about/index.html. Accessed 20 April 2013.

National Alliance for Caregiving and AARP (2009). *Caregiving in the U.S., 2009*. http://www.caregiving.org/pdf/research/caregivingusallagesexecsum.pdf. Accessed 10 April 2012.

Olmstead Act. (1999). Olmstead v. L. C. 527 U.S. 581 (1999). U.S. Supreme Court.

Olson, L. K. (Ed.). (1994). *The graying of the world: Who will care for the frail elderly*. New York: Haworth Press.

Ozawa, M. N., & Tseng, H. (1999). Utilization of formal services during the 10 years after retirement. *Journal of Gerontological Social Work, 31,* 3–20.

Patrick, J. H., & Goedereis, E. A. (2009). The importance of context and the gain-loss dynamic for understanding grandparent caregivers. In K. Shifren (Ed.), *How caregiving affects development: Psychological implications for child, adolescent, and adult caregivers* (pp. 169–190). Washington, DC: American Psychological Association.

Pavalko, E. K., & Woodbury, S. (2000). Social roles as process: Caregiving cases and women's health. *Journal of Health and Social Behavior, 41*(1), 91–105.

Perkins, E. A., & Haley, W. E. (2010). Compound caregiving: When lifelong caregivers undertake additional caregiving roles. *Rehabilitation Psychology, 55*(4), 409–417.

Shifren, K. (2008). Early caregiving: Perceived parental relations on current health and social support. *Journal of Adult Development, 15,* 160–168.

Shifren, K. (Ed.). (2009). Introduction: A life span perspective on caregiving. In K. Shifren (Ed.), *How caregiving affects development: Psychological implications for child, adolescent, and adult caregivers* (pp. 3–35). Washington, DC: American Psychological Association.

Super, N. (2002). *Who will be there to care? The growing gap between caregiver supply and demand. National Health Policy Forum background paper, January 23, 2002*. Washington, DC: The George Washington University.

Talley, R. C., & Crews, J. E. (2007). Framing the public health of caregiving. *American Journal of Public Health, 97*(2), 224–228.

Toseland, R., & McCallion, P. (1997). Trends in caregiving intervention research. *Social Work Research, 21,* 154–164.

U.S. Department of Health and Human Services (HHS) and U.S. Department of Labor (DOL) (2003). *The future supply of long-term care workers in relation to the aging baby boom generation: Report to Congress*. Washington, DC: Office of the Assistant Secretary for Planning and Evaluation. http://aspe.hhs.gov/daltcp/reports/ltcwork.htm. Accessed 21 March 2013.

U.S. Census Bureau (3 January 2006). Facts for feature. http://www.censusgov/Press-Release/www./releases/archives/facts_for_features_special-editions/006105html. Accessed 1 May 2012.

Wagner, D. L., & Niles, K. J. (2005). Looking into the future of family caregiving in the U.S. Proceedings from a White House conference on aging mini-conference, Convened 15 June 2005. http://www.towson.edu/healthscience/gerontology/documents/WHCA-Miniconf.pdf. Accessed 10 August 2010.

Wakabayashi, C., & Donato, K. M. (2006). Does caregiving increase poverty among women in later life? Evidence from the Health and Retirement Survey. *Journal of Health and Social Behavior, 47,* 258–274.

Chapter 2
Social Change and Caregiving

2.1 Introduction

Social change is a continuous process in all societies. Social change refers to any significant alteration over time in political, economic, social, and cultural institutions that result in changes in behavior patterns, cultural values, norms and beliefs. By "significant" sociologists mean changes resulting in profound and extensive societal consequences. Examples include the industrial revolution, the abolition of slavery, the feminist movement, the Civil Rights Act of 1964, and medical advancements leading to increased longevity. Social change results in changes in norms, role relationships, and the distribution of power and resources and affects the way individual members of society define situations.

The causes of social change are usually numerous, cumulative, and interrelated, for example, the rising costs of healthcare, government policy, and legislation to control costs. Social movements play a role in inspiring some members of society to bring about social change, while other members may resist change, especially when individuals with vested interests feel threatened by potential change. All social change has costs and benefits. As a society we are continually challenged to minimize the costs and maximize the benefits of social change (Institute for Health and Aging 1996).

2.2 Trends in Caregiving

From our early history, caregiving in the U.S. has focused around family, kin, and friend/neighbor support relationships (Levine 2004). Close personal ties were observed to govern primary group relationships while weaker ties characterized secondary group relationships. Urbanization and industrialization were thought to reduce the frequency of contact and level of support from kin. Rural residents were expected to have stronger interpersonal ties than urban residents (Glasgow 2000). However, several generations of rural-to-urban migration has changed expected patterns of intergenerational relationships among rural versus urban older residents.

J. G. Bruhn, H. M. Rebach, *The Sociology of Caregiving*,
Clinical Sociology: Research and Practice, DOI 10.1007/978-94-017-8857-1_2,

A study of general patterns of urban and rural social relationships found that people in nonmetropolitan networks had known each other longer and more of them were kin (Beggs et al. 1996). Other research has shown that there is strength in weak ties when they are networked (Granovetter 1973).

Anticipated problems of baby boomers during old age are likely to be shared by both urban and rural residents, with neither group having an advantage over the other in caregiving support. An aging society means not only fewer middle-aged adults to care for older people, but also fewer workers to support Social Security and other government entitlements that benefit older people. The challenge is to interface formal and informal caregiving networks so that they support each other (Glasgow 2000).

Caregiving has always been a universal experience of compassion and familial responsibility in American society, but due to the forces of social change, caregiving has become an essential and growing part of healthcare, long-term care, and social service policy-making. Family caregivers provide approximately 80% of all long-term services and support for family members and friends across the lifespan, yet they are the most neglected group in the health and long-term healthcare system (Feinberg et al. 2003; Feinberg 2004).

Caregiving in the United States has evolved from the closed communities evident among seventeenth century settlers where needs and obligations were clearly defined to the twenty-first century where we live in open networks of intimate associations and casual acquaintances, e.g. Facebook (Wuthnow 1991). Sociologist Robert Wuthnow (1998) has said that indifference, rather than caring, is the norm in twenty-first century America where kindness is a social problem because there is not enough of it. He explained, stating that the use and abuse of kindness in American life is not so much a matter of individual failings as it is the way our institutions operate. One of the effects of social change is that not all of our institutions react to change in the same way or at the same time. As a result, many of our institutions have "lagged" behind others and become porous and fragmented, altering the way we relate to one another and allow people to fall through the cracks (Wuthnow 1998). For example, the climate for human embryonic stem cell research in the U.S. is decidedly mixed. President George Bush stopped federal funding for new cell lines in stem cell research in the U.S. in 2001. States and private groups began funding stem cell research in 2004. In California Proposition 71 was approved to distribute several billion dollars in state funds to its universities and research institutions for stem cell research. Court challenges delayed the awarding of monies until 2006. Other states committed funds to counteract restrictive federal policies (Hampton 2006). By executive order on March 9, 2009, President Obama removed certain restrictions on federal funds involving new lines of human embryonic stem cells.

Wuthnow said, because of social changes such as increased diversity, fluidity, independence, and specialization of contemporary life, we favor short-term and sporadic commitments and task-specific relationships. In contrast to our founding fathers, we favor less rigid boundaries and caregiving activities that are loose networks of individuals who come together for a specific purpose such as volunteering, self-help groups, online groups and organizations, and nonkin networks.

Table 2.1 U.S. population, by age group: 1950–2050. (Source: Congressional Research Service 7-5700, March 31, 2011. www.crs.gov. Based on the Census Bureau's December 2010 data release. These data do not include results from the 2010 census)

Age/year	1950	1975	2000	2025	2050
Number (in thousands, rounded)					
Total	152,272	215,972	282,171	357,452	439,010
0–19	51,673	75,646	80,576	94,254	112,940
20–64	88.202	117,630	166,522	199,290	237,523
65–65+	12,397	22,696	35,074	63,907	88,547
Percent in Age Group (rounded)					
0–19	33.9	35.0	28.6	26.4	25.7
20–64	57.9	54.5	59.0	55.8	54.1
65–65+	8.1	10.5	12.4	17.9	20.2

2.3 An Aging Society and Caregiving

A recent report prepared for members of the U.S. Congress stated that "The U.S. is getting bigger, older, and more diverse" (Shrestha and Heisler 2011). Since 1950 the U.S. has experienced rapid population aging. (See Table 2.1.) The population growth is due to the trends of increased births, decreased deaths, increased immigration and increased longevity. The aging of the population is reflected in the proportion of persons aged 65 and over and an increasing median age of the population.

Indeed, the fastest growing age group in the U.S. is age 85 and over (See Fig. 2.1).

Immigration has had an effect on the size and age structure in the population. The increase in ethnic older adults is a significant factor in the aging population. By 2050, 39 % of the nation's older adults will be from minority groups. Cultural differences based on attitudes, beliefs, and behaviors are passed on from one generation to another and are important in caregiving.

Finally, scientific achievements have greatly alleviated the effects of many infectious diseases. The development of vaccines, effective mosquito control, and the introduction of modern sanitation has rendered diseases like polio, yellow fever, malaria, and cholera unheard of in the U.S. As a result, life expectancy in the U.S. has risen from 47 years in 1900 to 78.3 years in 2010.

The aging of the U.S. population will have increasing effects on health and healthcare services due to the increased numbers of persons experiencing some type of health condition. As the U.S. population ages, the social and economic demands on individuals, families, communities and the government will grow with effects on the formal and informal health and social service systems and on the financing of healthcare in general.

In conjunction with the growing numbers of older persons, the U.S. faces changes in the rates and outcomes of various conditions and disabilities. Trends in cognitive impairment and dementia have large policy implications for long-term institutional care. The use of long-term care is expected to increase the longer people live (Shrestha and Heisler 2011). Nearly three quarters of long-term care expenses are currently funded by public programs such as Medicaid. The estimated cost of Alzheimer's disease to Medicare and Medicaid totaled $ 50 billion in 2000

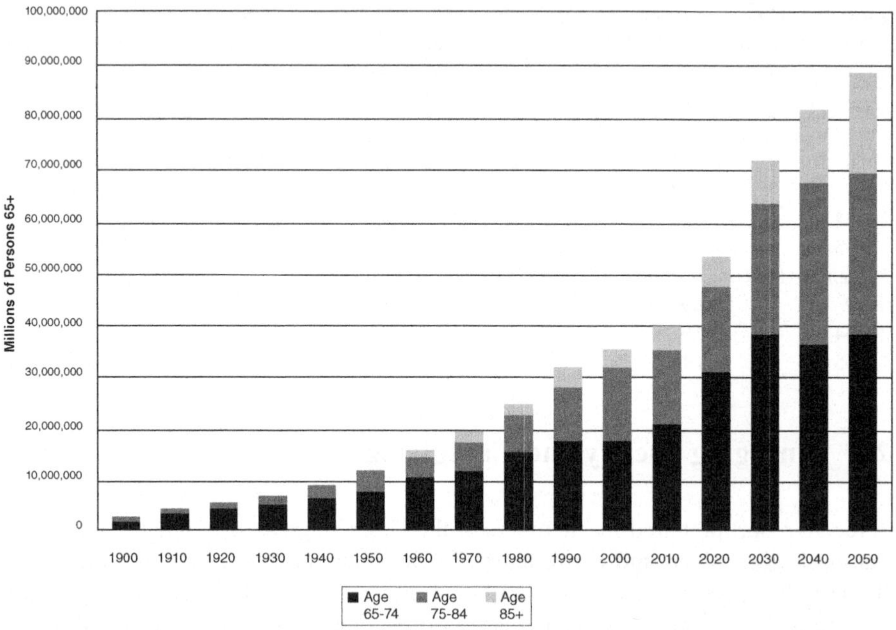

Fig. 2.1 U.S. population 65+ by age: 1900–2050. (Source: Projections of the population by age and sex for the United States: 2010 to 2050 (NP2008-T12), population division, U.S. census. Populations by age and sex for the United States: 1990 to 2000, part A. Number, Hobbs, Frank and Nicole Stoops, U.S. Census Bureau, special reports, series CENSR-4, demographic trends in the twentieth century. Compiled by the U.S. Administration on aging using the census data noted)

and is projected to be $ 200 billion by 2012 (Alzheimer's Association 2012). (See Fig. 2.2). Furthermore, questions arise as to the best ways to organize, access, and deliver services to older adults who have limited financial resources.

Immigration issues also have implications for policy. Pursuing an immigration strategy that favors workers entering for employment reasons may slow U.S. population aging therefore averting or delaying some policy challenges. Immigration may also create a number of policy challenges. For example, immigrants overly concentrated in certain geographic areas may strain local government infrastructure and resources.

Along with increased immigration there are increases in interethnic and interracial marriage, which has led to a growing multiracial population. This diversity presents policy and service challenges in a number of areas especially assimilation, income disparities, and poverty. In addition, there are differences in how different ethnic and racial groups use health services. It is essential that caregivers be cognizant of cultural differences among care recipients and their families and tailor expectations and behaviors with respect to ethnic beliefs and values. Caregivers need to understand the value system of elders and assess the extent to which care recipients hold on to traditional values. There are also differences in the types of care sought and utilized by race and ethnicity, differences in health conditions experienced, and differences in mortality rates for specific conditions (Shrestha and Heisler 2011).

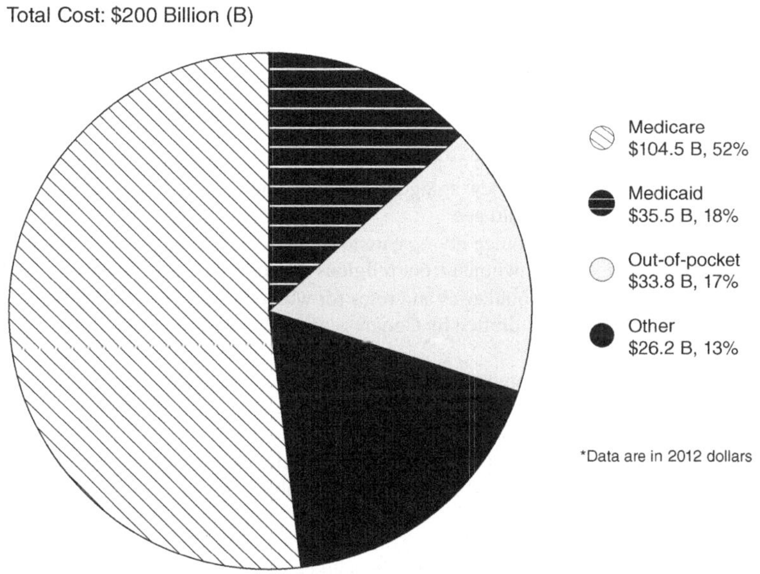

Fig. 2.2 Aggregate costs of care by payer for Americans age 65 and older with Alzheimer's disease and other dementias 2012*. (Source: Alzheimer's Association 2012, Alzheimer's disease facts and figures)

These differences could mean that some groups will experience poorer health and a greater need for caregiving resources at certain ages. Lehman (2009) pointed out, caregivers need to take into consideration the national origin of care recipients, age and gender, and the level of acculturation especially when the cultural origin of the caregiver differs from that of the care recipient. Caregivers' cultural backgrounds can also influence the relationship between caregivers' support networks and their personal strain as well as coping strategies.

The effect of a changing age structure will create new and broad changes in American life. According to Kass (2005) we will live differently, work differently, and think differently in a society in which the needs of the old become more dominant.

2.3.1 The Effects of Gender, Rights and Equality Issues on Caregiving

Forces shaping the evolution of gender, rights, and equality issues can be understood historically by examining three models for organizing work and family: *the household economy model, the dual breadwinner/female caregiver model, and the male breadwinner/female caregiver model* (Boris and Lewis 2006). The household economy model was evident in Colonial America, followed by the male breadwinner/female caregiver model in the nineteenth century, and the dual breadwinner/female caregiver model in the twentieth century. These models overlap in their evolution rather than follow a linear chronology. Table 2.2 shows how major themes of

Table 2.2 Major themes of caregiving during different eras in U.S. history. (Time periods and historical eras accessed from http://www.U-S-history.com/pages/eras.html)

Historical era	Major theme of caregiving
To 1630 Early America	Simple, direct, informal, technologically and knowledge-limited, family-focused
1630–1763 The colonial period	Women as primary caregivers, home-based care, low life expectancy, aging parents used contracts to guarantee their support in old age
1763–1783 Revolutionary America	Women giving care to soldiers in their homes and field hospitals, women from religious orders giving care to soldiers
1783–1815 The young republic, first industrial revolution	Boundaries and roles for women debated; a Bill of Rights was drafted by Congress and submitted to the states
1815–1860 Expansion, political reform, turmoil	Domestic slaves used as caregivers, reform of mental hospitals and use of caregivers
1830–1876 Sectional controversy, civil war, reconstruction	Social obligation of reciprocity to guarantee care in old age, first nurse training school established
1871–1914 Second industrial revolution	Germ theory of disease improved public health and sanitation, reduced infection and death, life expectancy 48 years
1880–1920 Political reform II	Healthcare moved to hospitals; women's political movements
1914–1933 World War I, prosperity, depression	Women enter workforce in great numbers, women veterans as caregivers; disabled veterans with chronic care needs; licensing of group child care homes
1933–1945 The silent generation, World War II	Traumatic stress disorder appears; Holocaust experiences of survivors
1945–1960 Postwar America Korean war	Studies of caregiving contexts; Migration away from parents and families, population of 65 and over increasing; many baby boomers are caregivers for spouses
1960–1980 The Vietnam era, civil rights	Studies of role strain and role conflict; 60 % of older Americans lived at or near poverty, 80 % relied solely on Social Security; end of life issues, the care of HIV/AIDS patients
1980–2000 End of twentieth century, Persian Gulf war	Advent of hospice in U.S., importance of patient's culture in caregiving; Alzheimer's and dementia major problems; women represent one half of workforce.
2001– The new millennium, Iraq-Afghanistan wars, terrorism, economic downturn	Care in institutional settings more common, but at high cost, care given by a network of providers; group homes common; Veteran's Care Act of 2005; working caregivers; Patient's Bill of Rights

caregiving have evolved and changed during different eras in U.S. history from the Colonial Period to the present day to the twenty-first century.

2.3.2 The Household Economy Model

During Colonial America work and family life was organized so that all members of the household shared responsibility for household maintenance. Men took responsibility for most tasks outside the home while women worked largely within the home preparing meals, laundering, cleaning, and caring for children. Women also joined neighbors to assist at sickbeds, weddings and funerals. Some women worked as professional midwives and provided social support in times of need. Women's roles overlapped and continued this way throughout the nineteenth and into the twentieth centuries. Men were heads of households and of their communities. Women's work was highly valued and while they were not seen or treated as social, political or economic equals to their husbands, they were recognized as contributing valuable labor to their households (Boris and Lewis 2006).

Gender roles in America changed little in the early nineteenth century despite social changes that accompanied industrialization and urbanization. There was greater participation by women in farm work and in industrial work that produced goods for sale at the market and yielded earned wages. The household economy model also was followed by African American families throughout the nineteenth and early twentieth centuries.

After the Civil War, African Americans sought social, political, and economic independence. Freed women sought a balance between work and family responsibilities. The household economy model also held for immigrants coming to the U.S. during the late nineteenth and early twentieth centuries; the typical first generation immigrant family worked as a productive unit, yet women assumed responsibility for domestic duties, while men's efforts were primarily wage earning.

Family caregiving was the model in the United States during its colonization by European settlers in the latter part of the eighteenth century (Manring et al. 2009; Scharlach 2008; Tanielian and Jaycock 2008). Caring for sick family members was considered to be part of a woman's job. Almost all caregiving was done at home. Lacking formal knowledge of disease, women provided care based on their own personal experiences. It wasn't until the Civil War (1861–1865) that formal caregiving was established in the form of professional nursing in the United States (Domrose 2011).

When the Civil War broke out there were no military nurses and most caregiving duties were assigned to convalescing soldiers who were well enough to perform them and to women in religious orders who cared for soldiers on both sides (Egenes 2009). The Civil War soon became too large on both sides to limit women who were willing to work for the military. Some historical accounts estimate there were 2,000 nurses on each side. Union hospital documents show at least 21,000 women on the payroll. Some women volunteered with aid organizations or religious groups, others followed their husbands or brothers to the battlefields, still others were freed and escaped slaves.

Women cared for sick and wounded soldiers on the battlefields, in field hospitals, in hospitals away from battle sites, and even in their own homes. Many women, widowed and without income, worked as hospital or field camp relief workers. Their titles and pay varied according to race and social class. The work of Civil War "nurses" proved that women could provide excellent care for men they were not related to without damaging their reputations. The Union Army added a small corps of 100 female nurses who were trained by Dorothea Dix who was named Superintendent of Union Army nurses during the war, already famous as a reformer and advocate for the mentally ill, and Elizabeth Blackwell, the nation's first female physician.

The work and writings of Florence Nightingale, a British nurse, who elevated the role of caregiver to that of a professional nurse during the Crimean War in 1854 when she brought standards of care and infection control to wounded soldiers, became known in the U.S. Nightingale's teachings about sanitation proved helpful in preventing the spread of infection and disease, which killed more soldiers than wounds. A combination of Nightingale's work, advances in medicine, and growth of hospitals, and the inspiration of Civil War nursing stories created a climate for professional nursing education. The U.S. Sanitary Commission lobbied for the establishment of the country's first nursing schools in New York, Connecticut, and Massachusetts (Larson 1997).

2.3.3 The Male Breadwinner/Female Caregiver Model

Urban industrialization in the mid-nineteenth century in America created a dramatic reorganization of home and work that developed a model with sharper distinctions between men's and women's work and family responsibilities. Men were clearly the economic providers; wages became a standard for manhood. Women's work that did not earn a wage was considered non-productive. Women's domestic labor was termed "care" rather than work. This transformed the meaning of domesticity especially among the middle class and among white women. As Boris and Lewis (2006) stated, "household work became invisible" p. 79.

Wage work that women engaged in outside the home was considered temporary and circumstantial. Women who were permanent wage earners were disparaged because they were unable to live up to fulfilling their domestic role as caregivers. Women's work was not given the same value as a man's. This point of view extended to all women including immigrants. Women, especially those from the educated middle-class, increasingly sought work outside the home and initiated social reforms. They called for public recognition to legitimatize their work. Women's work became regarded as failed responsibility of men to support their families economically.

Some mothers delayed entry into the work force until their children started school. For others childcare became an issue. Some middle-class reformers established day care nurseries to help poor wage-earning mothers. Mothers' petitions of the 1910s and 1920s evolved into Aid to Dependent Children (ADC) under Social Security in 1935.

The New Deal in the 1930s institutionalized the country's commitment to the male breadwinner/female caregiver model as the appropriate relationship between men and women. Relief programs such as the Works Progress Administration (WPA) reinforced gender and racial hierarchies by employing men over women and whites over other groups. Programs under the New Deal linked work to benefits so that some people would get benefits by virtue of their gender or paid employment. Aid to Dependent Children (ADC) also became a means-tested stimatized program which was run by the states and varied greatly in requirements and amount of aid. During World War II the federal government increased child-care funding for wage-earning mothers, most working mothers found other forms of child care.

Some corporations and industries reimbursed employed mothers for meals and laundry to ease their burden. By the end of World War II the male breadwinner model/female caregiver model was institutionalized in public programs and in cultural expectations.

2.3.4 The Dual Breadwinner/Female Caregiver Model

Post-World War II social policies encouraged mothers to enter the labor force and work overtime while fulfilling their family and domestic responsibilities. The 1950s were recognized by historians as a period of wage-earner mothers, overlapping models for combining work and family. Nonetheless, the male breadwinner remained the ideal, with whites as the norm. Only during the 1960s did the rights movement come to dominate discussions of women and employment (Boris and Lewis 2006). With half of the employed women married and a third of married wage earners with children under age 18 in 1953, the U.S. Women's Bureau sought to improve the income, benefits, hours, and working conditions of women wage earners. The President's Commission on the Status of Women, created by John F. Kennedy in 1961, had as its task to recommend ways to overcome discrimination in government and private employment on the basis of sex, but also enable women to continue their roles as wives and mothers while making a contribution to the world around them. Women tended to see themselves as workers and mothers, breadwinners and homemakers; they refused to choose breadwinning over caregiving or equate equality with assimilation to the male sphere (Boris and Lewis 2006). The public agenda also ignored how women from other racial and ethnic groups managed to combine work and family.

The Civil Rights Act of 1964 was a landmark piece of legislation in the U.S. that outlawed major forms of discrimination against African-Americans and women, including racial segregation. It ended unequal application of voter registration requirements and racial segregation in schools, in the workplace, and in facilities that served the general public. Among some of the first complaints filed by the Equal Employment Opportunity Commission (EEOC), the federal agency formed to administer the law, were charges of pregnancy discrimination. It was claimed that management forced pregnant mothers to quit their jobs, took away their seniority, or deprived them of sickness and accident benefits. The Pregnancy Discrimination Act (PDA) of 1978 held that pregnancy would be treated not as a disability but in terms of its comparability with other conditions that impacted employment. After the PDA labor unions, for example, could negotiate paid pregnancy leave and non-paid child-care leave with large employers and airlines permitted flight attendants to apply sick leave to pregnancy rather than terminating them. State laws offered other treatments for pregnancy.

The Family and Medical Leave Act (FMLA), introduced in 1985, became law in 1993; it permitted men and women, in companies with 50 or more employees, 3 months of unpaid leave for birth, adoption, or care of an ill family member and

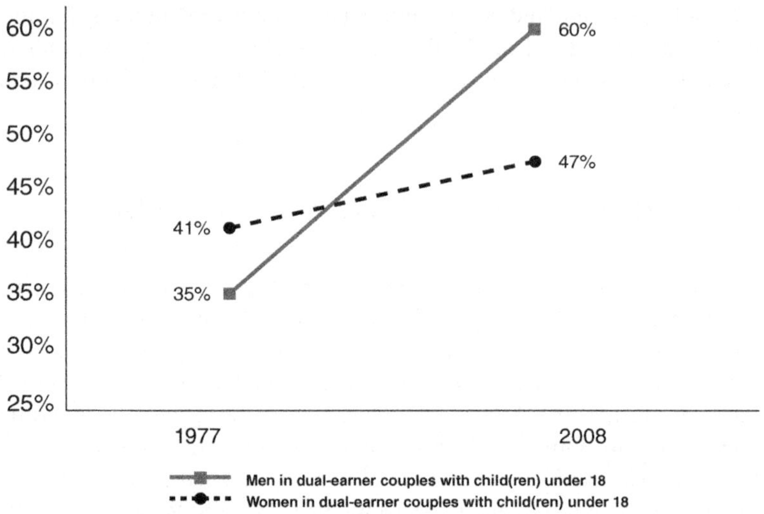

Statistically significant differences between men and women in dual-earner couples with children under 18: 1977 not significant; 2008 p<.01; Statistically significant differences between 1977 and 2008: Men p<.001; women not significant. Sample size: 1977 n=283: 2008 n=391.

Fig. 2.3 Percentage of fathers and mothers in dual-earner couples reporting work-family conflict (1977–2008). (Source: 2008 NSCW, FWI and 1977 QES, U.S. Department of Labor)

the leave taken was with guaranteed job and health benefits.[1] The Act was seen as having the potential of providing relief to women who face the stressful demands of multiple roles (Jenkins 1997).

In the period since the FMCA Act the conventions about what it means to be a man in today's workplaces and families have changed. Traditional gender roles have become more egalitarian and challenging. Surveys have found that this change has not been easy for men to adjust to (Galinsky et al. 2009). A man today is someone who is not only successful as a financial provider but is also involved as a father, husband/partner and son. Men who work long hours in demanding jobs and are work-centric or are fathers in dual-earner households, are at-risk for work-family conflict. Men are now experiencing what women found when they first entered the workforce—the pressure to do it all and have it all (Thomas 2012). See Fig. 2.3. Aumann et al. (2011) suggest that change needs to occur in individual attitudes about work and family and workplace design as well as cultural change that dispels the mystiques for both men and women.

When men and women both experience more equality in the workplace in terms of pay and career advancement opportunities they will have choices in how they can better manage breadwinning and caregiving roles.

[1] Since the passage of the Family and Medical Leave Act (FMLA) in 1993, 21 states have dropped the family component of the original law and, instead, reduced coverage to baby care or parental leave. This shifts the emphasis on family, including care of elderly parents, to parental, baby care only. With the baby boom population aging the demand for family care will increase and employers will be pressured by employees for release time to assist aging parents. See Wisensale (2003).

2.4 Effects of Changes in Disease Types and Lifestyles on Caregiving

The twentieth century was characterized by profound changes that have influenced how we live including changes in the patterns and distribution of disease. Many interdependent factors helped to create these changes which are woven into multi-dimensional networks. Today's diseases are very different than they were a century ago. Changes in the physical and social environments, new technologies, and advances in public health and in medicine, have all contributed to a higher proportion of the population now living to old age.

In the twentieth century, life expectancy in developed countries increased at the rate of 2 to 3 years added to life with each decade that has passed. The increase in life expectancy was accompanied by an "epidemiological transition" characterized by a shift from acute infections and deficiency diseases to chronic non-communicable diseases.[2] The most evident indicators of this transition are changes in the pattern of mortality as well as changes in morbidity. This shift was not a linear, smooth process, but a complex, dynamic, uneven, and sometimes unpredictable result of demographic, economic, technological, social and cultural factors that have appeared, disappeared, and reappeared over time. Figure 2.4 shows the shifts in the leading causes of death from 1900 to 1990. Chronic diseases, whose causes are largely linked to lifestyle, are predominant.

Social change, directly and/or indirectly, is involved in the epidemiological transition. Social, cultural, behavioral, and technological factors are closely linked (Wahdan 1996). The shift from an agricultural to an industrial society and its accompanying process of modernization has produced changes that have influenced people's health. For example, regular exercise has been shown to have health benefits. Exercise levels are a matter of individual choice but are influenced by competing time demands and accessibility. People who live in neighborhoods that lack social cohesion or sidewalks that are considered safe, limit their exercise, and have been shown to be at risk for depression and obesity. Suburban spread has contributed to a decline in exercise and a greater dependence on cars. Sprawl, television, computers, and the Internet also can contribute to social isolation. We have shifted from being a more communal society to an individualistic one.

One of the key risk factors brought to prominence by social and lifestyle changes is the growing epidemic of obesity among American adults and children. It is predicted that 42% of the U.S. population could be obese by 2030. One concern is how many of today's obese children will grow up to be obese adults. According to the Centers for Disease Control and Prevention (CDC) more than one-third of U.S. adults (35.7%) are obese. By state, the prevalence of obesity ranges from a low of 21% in Colorado to a high of 34.0% in Mississippi in 2010. The South has the highest prevalence of obesity followed by the Midwest, Northeast and the West. Figure 2.5 shows the prevalence of obesity throughout the U.S. in 2010.

---

[2] M. Schulman pointed to 12 key diseases whose control has altered history. They are: smallpox, tuberculosis, syphilis, HIV/AIDS, influenza, bubonic plague, cholera, malaria, yellow fever, hemophilia and porphyria, and plant disease. See Schulman (2008).

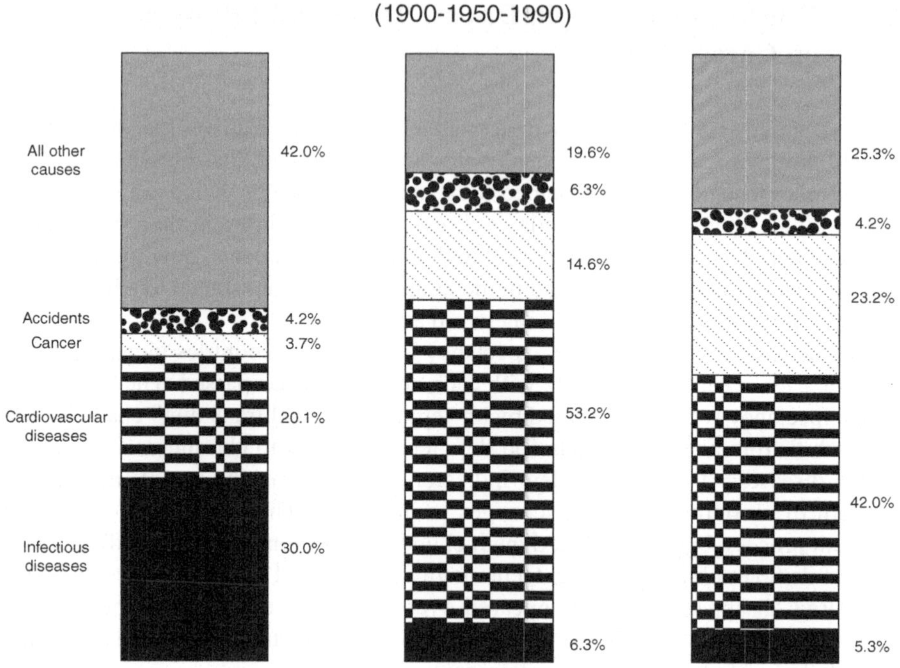

Fig. 2.4 Changes in leading causes of death. (Source: U.S. Bureau of the census, statistical abstract of the United States, 1993 (113th edition), Washington, D.C. 1993 (1980–1990). U.S. Bureau of the census, Historical abstracts of the United States, colonial times to 1970, bicentennial edition, part 1, Washington, D.C. 1993 (1980–1990))

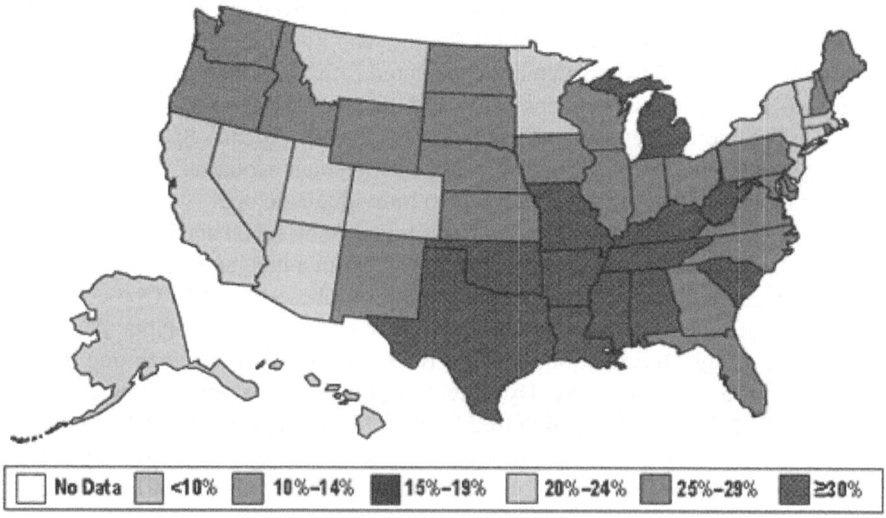

Fig. 2.5 Percentage of obesity (BMI > 30) in U.S. adults, 2010. (Source: Center for Disease Control and Prevention)

Table 2.3 Actual causes of death in the United States in 1990 and 2000. (Source: Mokdad et al. 2004)

Actual cause	No. (%) in 1990	No. (%) in 2000
Tobacco	400,000 (19)	435,000 (18.1)
Poor diet and physical inactivity	300,000 (14)	400,000 (16.6)
Alcohol consumption	100,000 (5)	85,000 (3.5)
Microbial agents	90,000 (4)	75,000 (3.1)
Toxic agents	60,000 (3)	55,000 (2.3)
Motor vehicle	25,000 (1)	43,000 (1.8)
Firearms	35,000 (2)	29,000 (1.2)
Sexual behavior	30,000 (1)	20,000 (0.8)
Illicit drug use	20,000 (< 1)	17,000 (0.7)
Total	*1,060,000 (50)*	*1,159,000 (48.2)*

Obesity is a risk factor for several chronic diseases including diabetes, heart disease and cancer. Consequently these diseases may result in disability and the need for long-term care. The financial costs of obesity-related illnesses is said to approach $ 190.2 million annually (McKay 2012).

2.5 Social Change and Risk Factors for Disease

We are all daily, life-long participants in social change. Social change frequently forces us to make choices about our lives as individuals or as members of families, communities or a society. Choices entail varying degrees of risk-taking; some risks have consequences that may not be known for decades. Such is the case with choices we make regarding our health behavior. We make our choices in an environment of constant change. We feel less risky about the choices we make about health behavior when the observations and experiences of others affirm our own beliefs and experiences. Making choices about health habits is more often unfortunately learned by trial and error than taught as part of our socialization. Looking at the actual causes of death in the U.S. for 1990 and 2000 indicates that there are modifiable risk factors associated with many of the actual causes of death in the U.S. (Table 2.3).

The actual causes of death in 1990 and 2000 were tobacco (19 %), poor diet and physical inactivity (14 %), and alcohol consumption (5 %). Other actual causes of death were microbial agents (4 %), toxic agents (3 %), motor vehicle crashes (1 %), incidents involving firearms (2 %), sexual behavior (1 %), and illicit drug use (< 1 %) (Mokdad et al. 2004). These findings, along with escalating healthcare costs and an aging population, argue for the need for a more preventive orientation among the U.S. population. About half of all deaths that occurred in the U.S. in 1990 and 2000 could be attributed to a large number of preventable behaviors.[3] The most striking finding was the substantial increase from 1990 to 2000 in the number of deaths due to poor diet and physical inactivity.

[3] Also see National Center for Health Statistics (2011).

A group of researchers estimated how much risk each of 12 modifiable risk factors from national health surveys contributed to premature or preventable deaths. Modifiable risk factors fell into three main groups. There were lifestyle risk factors such as tobacco smoking, physical inactivity, and excessive alcohol use. A second group was dietary risk factors such as high salt intake and low intake of fruits and vegetables. A third group was comprised of metabolic risk factors that increased cardiovascular disease and diabetes. They concluded that these factors can be influenced by individual level and population-wide interventions. In particular, effective interventions are available for tobacco smoking and high blood pressure, two leading causes of death in the U.S. Despite the availability of interventions, blood pressure and tobacco smoking decline in the U.S. have stagnated and even reversed and there has been a steady increase in overweight-obesity. These risk factors have serious implications for caregiving needs currently and in the future (Danaei et al. 2009).

2.6 Implications for Caregiving

While medical care and prevention efforts have contributed to increases in life expectancy in the U.S. during the past century, they have also produced a major shift in the leading causes of death for all age groups, including older adults. In 2002 the top three causes of death for U.S. adults aged 65 and older were heart disease, cancer, and stroke. These accounted for 61 % of all deaths in this age group (Fig. 2.6).

The tragedy is that heart disease, cancer, and stroke are often preventable. Although the risk for disease and disability increase with age, poor health is not an inevitable consequence of aging. These behaviors—smoking, poor diet, and physical inactivity—were the root causes of almost 35 % of U.S. deaths in 2000 (Centers for Disease Control and Prevention 2007). These behaviors often underlie the development of heart disease, cancer, stroke and diabetes.

Death is only part of the picture of the burden of chronic diseases among older Americans. These conditions can cause years of pain, disability, loss of function and independence before ending in death. Currently, at least 80 % of older Americans are living with one chronic condition, 50 % have two. (See Fig. 2.7)

The nation's healthcare costs continue to rise. The cost of providing healthcare for one person aged 65 and older is three to five times greater than the cost to someone younger than 65. This is because of the need for costs getting to care, receiving assistance, and usually the treatment is more complex and extended. By 2030, healthcare spending will increase by 25 % largely because the population will be older. This is without consideration of inflation costs and the higher cost of improved medical technology. Medicare spending alone has increased nine-fold over the past two decades from $ 37 billion in 1980 to $ 336 billion in 2005 (Centers for Disease Control and Prevention 2007).

Caregiving today is much more challenging than it was in the past and those challenges are likely to grow even more daunting in the future (Kass 2007). The sick and elderly are likely to have multiple illnesses requiring different kinds of care

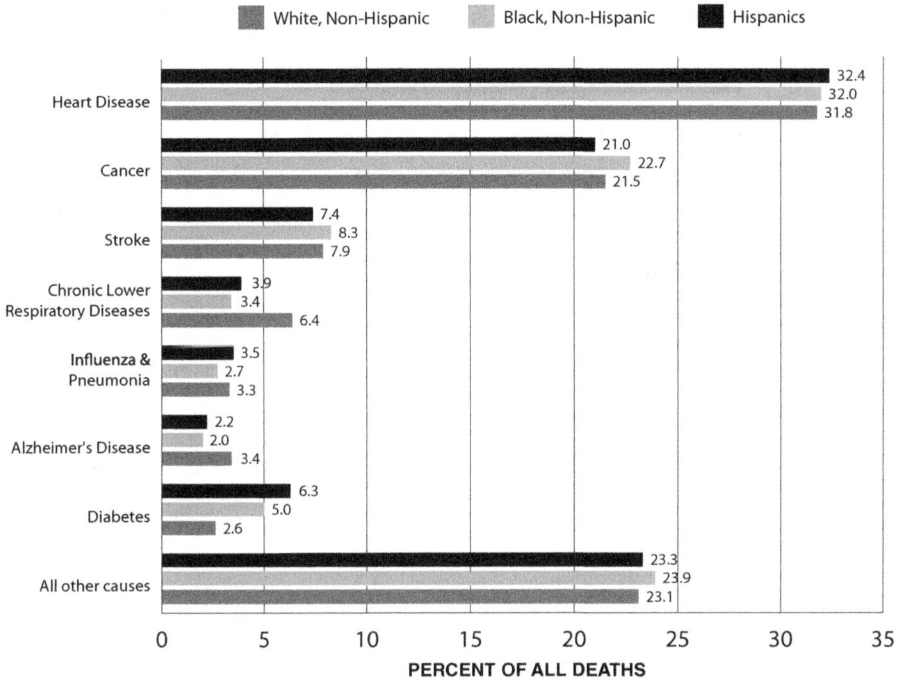

Fig. 2.6 Chronic diseases were the leading causes of death among U.S. adults aged 65 or in 2002. (Source: CDC, National Center for Health Statistics. National Vital Statistics System, 2006)

for longer periods of time since elderly and frail patients frequently survive longer than in the past. Families are smaller so elderly patients have fewer family members to rely on for care. The typical family caregiver in the past was a woman who didn't work outside the home. Now working women caregivers spend as long in adult caregiving as they do in caring for children. Sometimes the use of paid caregivers is only temporary or short-term because of limited financial or insurance resources. The fluidity of caregiving requires caregivers to be continually vigilant for safety concerns and changes in the care recipient's condition.

2.7 Summary

Social change is inevitable in human societies. We create some change, other change obccurs naturally. Change in demographics, gender equality and workforce patterns, medical technology, preventive medicine and economics are some of the factors that have changed family caregiving. The U.S. population is aging and people are living longer, which also means years of illness, disability, and dependence. While the majority of long-term care is still provided at home by family members, as the needs of more Americans become more complex, intensive, and demanding, there

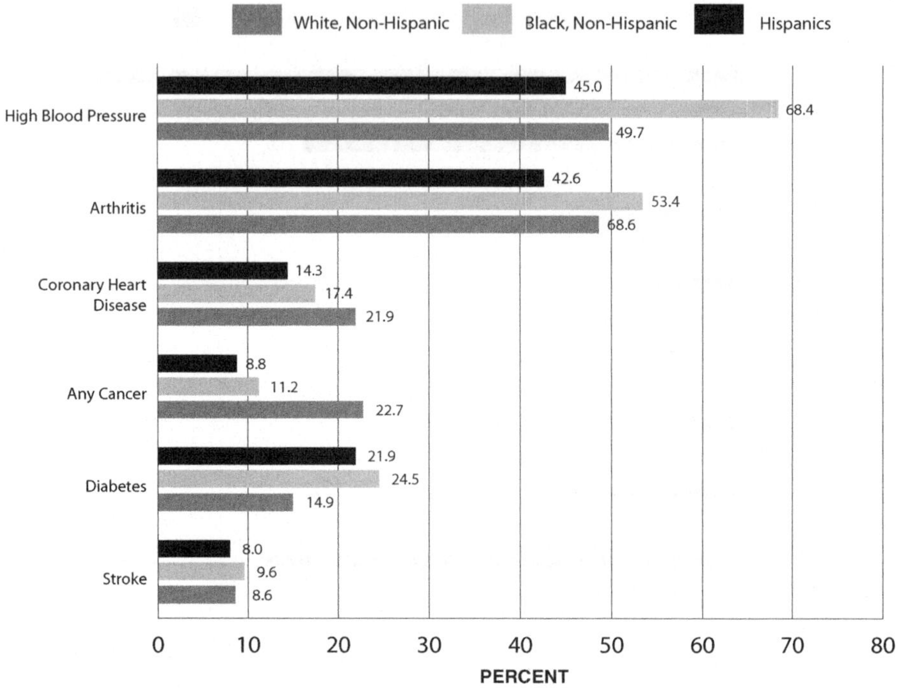

Fig. 2.7 Prevalence of chronic conditions among adults aged 65 years or older varied by race/ethnicity in 2002–2003. (Source: CDC, National Center for Health Statistics. National Health Interview Survey, 2006)

is an increasing need for more paid and volunteer caregivers. Women, who have been the traditional family caregivers, are now in the paid workforce and only 40 % of all adult caregivers are men. Family caregivers are often expected to provide the level of care that only a few decades ago was reserved for hospitals, but they are not trained to carry out some tasks. There is an increasing shortage of trained caregivers to meet the needs of our population over age 65. Changes in family structure have not lessened the need for people to care for others, but healthcare, legal and policy systems in the U.S. have not kept up with social change.[4]

2.8 Questions for Discussion

1. What are some of the lessons learned from recent wounded survivors of war about their long-term care needs?

[4] See Levine (2008).

2. There have been recent efforts by many states to drop paid family leave from the original Family and Medical Leave Act of 1993, which shifts the emphasis on family (including care of elderly parents) to parental care (baby care only). Discuss the implications of this considering the growing aging population that will demand greater assistance from family caregivers and in need of benefits such as family leave.
3. How do you see the future need for caregivers being met?
4. Caregiving is a total commitment. You never feel like you do enough. What are factors to consider whether or not there is a need for professionals to begin to provide care for your family member?
5. What do you consider to be the key factors that continue to influence the nature of caregiving in the U.S.?

References

Alzheimer's Association (2012). Facts and Figures. https://www.alz.org/downloadsfacts_figures_2012.pdf. Accessed 10 January 2014.

Aumann, K., Galinsky, E., & Matos, K. (2011). *The new male mystique*. New York: Families and Work Institute.

Beggs, S., Haines, V. A., & Hurlbert, J. S. (1996). Revisiting the rural-urban contrast: Personal networks in nonmetropolitan and metropolitan settings. *Rural Sociology, 61*(2), 306–325.

Boris, E., & Lewis, C. H. (2006). Caregiving and wage-earning: A historical perspective on work and family. In M. Pitt-Catsouphes, E. E. Kossek, & S. Sweet (Eds.), *The work and family handbook: Multi-disciplinary perspectives, methods, and approaches* (pp. 73–87). Mahwah: Lawrence Erlbaum.

Centers for Disease Control and Prevention and the Merck Company Foundation (2007). The state of aging in America, 2007. Whitehouse Station, NJ. The Merck Company Foundation. www.cdc.gov/aging and www.merck.com/cr. Accessed 10 June 2013.

Danaei, G., Ding, E. L., Mozaffarian, O., Taylor, B., Rehm, J., Murray, C. J. L., & Ezzati, M. (2009). The preventable causes of death in the United States: Comparative risk assessment of dietary, lifestyle, and metabolic risk factors. *PLoS Medicine, 6*(4), e1000058. doi:10.1371/journal.pmed.1000058.

Domrose, C. (29 April 2011). The civil war and nursing. http://news.nurse.com/article/20110429/NATIONAL01/304290019/-/frontpage. Accessed 25 April 2012.

Egenes, K. J. (2009). History of nursing. In G. Roux & J. A. Halstead (Eds.), *Issues and trends in nursing: Essential knowledge for today and tomorrow* (pp. 1–26). Sudbury: Jones & Bartlett Publishers.

Feinberg, L. F. (2004). Caregiving on the public policy agenda. In C. Levine (Ed.), *Always on call: When illness turns families into caregivers* (pp. 193–207). Nashville: Vanderbilt University Press.

Feinberg, L. F., Horvath, J., Hunt, G., Plooster, L., Kagan, J., Levine, C., Lynn, J., Mintz, S., & Wilkinson, A. (1 December 2003). Family caregiving and public policy principles for change. http://www.caregiving.org/data/principles04.pdf. Accessed 10 July 2010.

Galinsky, E., Aumann, K., & Bond, J. T. (2009). *Times are changing: Gender and generation at work and at home*. New York: Families and Work Institute. http://familiesandwork.org/site/research/reports/Times_Are_Changing.pdf. Accessed 10 June 2013.

Glasgow, N. (2000). Rural/urban patterns of aging and caregiving in the United States. *Journal of Family Issues, 21,* 611–631.

Granovetter, M. S. (1973). The strength of weak ties. *American Journal of Sociology, 78*(6), 1360–1380.
Hampton, T. (2006). U.S. cell research lagging. *Journal of the American Medical Association, 295*(19), 2233.
Institute for Health and Aging, University of California, San Francisco, CA. (1996). *Chronic care in America: A 21st century challenge*. Princeton: The Robert Wood Johnson Foundation. (publications@rwjf.org). Accessed 10 June 2013.
Jenkins, C. L. (1997). Women, work, and caregiving: How do these roles affect women's well-being. *Journal of Women & Aging, 9*(3), 27–45.
Kass, L. R. (2005). *Taking care: Ethical caregiving in our aging society*. Washington, DC: The President's Council on bioethics.
Larson, R. D. (1997). *White roses: Stories of civil war nurses*. Gettysburg: Thomas.
Lehman, D. (2009). 21st century caregivers: Diversity in culture. *Aging Well,* 2 (March-April) p. 26.
Levine, C. (Ed.) (2004). Introduction: The many worlds of family caregivers. In C. Levine (Ed.), *Always on call: When illness turns families into caregivers* (pp. 1–19). Nashville: Vanderbilt University Press.
Levine, C. (2008). Family caregiving. The Hastings Center. http://www.thehastingscenter.org/Publications/BriefingBook/Detail.aspx?id=2172. Accessed 22 March 2012.
Manring, M. M., Hawk, A., Calhoun, J. H., & Anderson, R. C. (2009). Treatment of war wounds: A historical review. *Clinical Orthopaedics and Related Research, 467*(8), 2168–2191.
McKay, B. (2012). The ABCs of beating obesity. *The Wall Street Journal,* (9 May).
Mokdad, A. H., Marks, J. S., Stroup, D. F., & Gerberding, J. L. (2004). Actual causes of death in the United States, 2000. *Journal of the American Medical Association, 291*(10), 1238–1245.
National Center for Health Statistics. (2011). *Health, United States, 2010: With special feature on death and dying*. Hyattsville: U.S. Department of Health and Human Services, Centers for Disease Control and Prevention. (DHHS Pub. No. 2011–1232).
Scharlach, A. (2008). Historical overview: Lessons from the past, challenges for the future in family caregiving. *American Journal of Nursing, 108*(9 Suppl), 16–22.
Schulman, M. (2008) 12 diseases that altered history. U.S. News & World Report, January 3.
Shrestha, L. B., & Heisler, E. J. (2011). The changing demographic profile of the United States. Congressional Research Service 7-5700. www.crs.gov. Accessed 31 March 2001.
Tanielian, T., & Jaycock, L. H. (Eds.). (2008). *Invisible wounds of war: Psychological and cognitive injuries, their consequences, and services to assist recovery*. Washington, DC: Rand Corporation. (Monograph MG-720).
Thomas, S. G. (2012). Are dads the new moms? *The Wall Street Journal,* (May 12–13).
Wahdan, M. H. (1996). The epidemiological transition. *Eastern Mediterranean Health Journal, 2*(1), 8–20.
Wisensale, S. K. (2003). Two steps forward, one step back: The Family and Medical Leave Act as retrenchment policy. *Review of Policy Research, 20*(1), 135–151.
Wuthnow, R. (1991). *Acts of compassion: Caring for others and helping ourselves*. Princeton: Princeton University Press.
Wuthnow, R. (1998). *Loose connections: Joining together in America's fragmented communities*. Cambridge: Harvard University Press.

Chapter 3
The Life Course Perspective

The life course perspective is a framework that has emerged over the past five or six decades within the social and behavioral sciences. It connects individual development with the social structure and culture as well as the historical time in which the stages of an individual's life take place. George (1993) asserted that the "life course is a social phenomenon, distinct from the life span. The life course reflects the intersection of social and historical factors with personal biography." She defined life-span simply as the duration of life.

Elder (1974; 1975) was one of the early sociologists to write about the life course perspective. He was prompted by his long-term studies of people who grew up during the Great Depression of the 1930s and his observations of the influence of social and historical forces on individual development (Hutchinson 2008).

Crosnoe and Elder (2002) observed that aging is a lifelong process. They studied aging with a sample of men who had participated in the Stanford-Terman study, a longitudinal study that began in 1922 that included periodic interviews and life history records. Their study used 424 men who were still alive in the 1970s and were contacted in 1972 and 1977. As the authors noted, the Terman study was a study of intellectually gifted children. The men in their sample were white Anglos from advantaged backgrounds who had achieved high levels of education.

Based on data from 1972 (the men were between age 58 and 67) and 1977 (ages 63 to 72), the authors created aging profiles based on four factors: (1) life satisfaction, (2) vitality, (3) family engagement, (4) occupational success, and (5) civic involvement. Cluster analysis was used which produced four general profiles or types, each of which illustrated different styles of aging. Detailed descriptions of these types are not relevant here, but what is relevant is how the types or styles of aging were the product of the interaction of current circumstances and life history. Life history may affect current circumstances, but, as Crosnoe and Elder concluded:

> … Lifelong experiences influence aging style in their own right by capturing the nature of the individual pathways through life, not simply by establishing current circumstances. In other words, knowledge of the journey supplements knowledge about the destination in explaining patterns of adjustment in the later years. (Crosnoe and Elder 2002)

Health in later life is critically related to the antecedent conditions and life course. As Pearlin et al. (2005) pointed out, stressors in earlier life stages have health ef-

J. G. Bruhn, H. M. Rebach, *The Sociology of Caregiving*,
Clinical Sociology: Research and Practice, DOI 10.1007/978-94-017-8857-1_3,

fects over time. People's positions in structures of inequality affect their exposure to stressors affecting health, well-being, and longevity. For example, the circumstances of a person's family of origin form a context in which exposure to health risk factors are more or less likely. These family-of-origin circumstances also affect a person's life chances for educational attainments and occupational and economic outcomes which further relate to health and longevity as well as quality of later aging.

Kahn and Pearlin (2006) noted that persistent and recurring stressors can lead to declining health. They also noted that health deficits caused by these stressors may develop slowly and have a cumulative effect which accelerates over the person's life course. Financial hardship is one such stressor. These researchers measured the timing and persistence of financial hardship over several stages of the life course of respondents, all over age 65 at the time of their study, to see if earlier financial stress was related to health later in life. They found that over half of their respondents reported financial hardships in childhood. This was consistent with the fact that the early years of these cohorts were spent during a time of economic depression. They also found that the percent of respondents reporting financial hardships declined after age 35, consistent with the economic expansion years of the late 1940s and 1950s. In addition, many in these cohorts would have benefited from legislation that created government education and housing programs as well as Social Security and Medicare.

With regard to timing, Kahn and Pearlin (2006) found that financial hardship in any of the life stages was associated with health outcomes in later life, even when such hardships were in childhood some 50 or more years earlier. And the effects on health increased when the financial hardship was present between ages 35 and 50 and continued to increase when financial stress occurred between ages 50 and 65. Finally, the results also showed that persistent economic hardship was more adverse than passing or episodic hardship, emphasizing the cumulative nature of these effects on health over the life course.

Closely related to health and certainly a part of psychological well-being is a person's sense of mastery. Pearlin et al. (2007) studied the life course conditions that promote mastery, person's sense of "their ability to manage the circumstances of their lives" (p. 164). Experiences over the life course including achievements and status attainments as well as exposure to stressors are proposed as antecedents to the level of mastery felt by the person. Data to test their model came from a sample of 1,167 respondents, 65 years of age and older, from the Washington, DC Metropolitan area drawn from Medicare files. Authors asserted that sampling this age group was especially suited to their purpose because, "at late life, it is possible to look for those antecedents of mastery that are spread across long periods of time and multiple segments of the life course" (p. 168). The expectation was that these elders' current level of mastery would be shaped by experiences over the life course.

Results showed that certain ascribed statuses, race and gender, "were significantly and independently related to mastery." Women and African Americans were less likely to express life course mastery. However, ascribed statuses became nonsignificant when status attainment was added to the analysis. Specifically, when educational achievement was added to the analysis, race and gender became non-significant. As the researchers commented, this showed that race and gender, as antecedents, create constraints (or enhancements) to life course opportunities. In this research educational achievement beyond high school accounted for the increase in mastery and was also associated with occupational attainment which also gave participants an enhanced sense of controlling the course of their lives.

When stressors and encountered hardships were added to the analysis, results showed that hardships and severe stressors tended to be greater among those with lower status attainment. Experiences of discrimination at work and/or at school as well as periods of economic hardship over the life course and recent experiences of caregiving were among stressors included. Results showed that the extent of these stressors over the life course was significantly and negatively related to level of mastery. But occupational prestige and accumulated wealth were related to mastery independent of the stressors and hardships assessed here. The authors interpreted this as: people's success or failure to reach desired goals has a basic influence on their sense of control of their life course trajectory regardless of the hardships and barriers they faced.

When recent stressors including caregiving were added to the analysis, only economic strain had an effect on participant's sense of mastery. Authors concluded that the sense of mastery is less a trait that some are endowed with and more a consequence that develops over the life course, based on antecedents related to ascribed statuses and the course of life's achievements. Particularly important were exposure to hardships and stressors that are resistant to personal control (Thoits 2006).

Crosnoe (2000) wrote that the life course perspective, "views lives as the enactment of a series of age-related roles that are embedded in socio-historical contexts." And Crosnoe and Elder (2002) emphasized, "Linking life stages, examining transitions, and exploring agency within context." The concept of linked lives calls our attention to the interdependence of people and the importance of shared relationships. For example, family members are linked and interdependent over time. There is continuity and change, for individuals and relationships.

Central to the life course perspective is the view that throughout the life course human lives are linked. Bruhn (2011) observed that humans need the support and companionship of others throughout their lives and that, "It is close social ties that give significance to individual lives." Interdependence across generations is a key feature of family life where members can find social, emotional, and material support from each other. The family represents and interprets the larger society to the child. Children learn the language, learn norms and values and important skills—become socialized—as they interact with family members. And the family can buffer aversive affects of social conditions presented by a neighborhood or the economic or social conditions of the society.

Family relationships develop over time, over stages of the life course, as people exchange social and emotional support and other reinforcers. Relationships between and among generations are an important source of support and emotional well-being. Antonucci et al. (2011) characterized intergenerational relationships as a "cornerstone of human interaction…." They referred to a *convoy model*, which suggests that persons travel through life surrounded by members of their convoy, others who provide help and support for growth and help facing life events. The various generations of one's family make up a key part of the convoy for many people. The form and quality of each of these relationships show cumulative development over time, across stages of the life course.

As children mature and become independent adults, the interdependence developed in earlier life stages continues. Relationships may serve as sources of affection and sense of belonging as well as sources of social support and social capital. When the need arises, care for older adults and family members with disabilities emerges out of the emotional bonds and concern for others' well-being formed and maintained across the stages of the life course.

Some form of reciprocity is at the heart of ongoing caregiving relationships. Emslie et al. (2009) studied spousal caregiving when one partner has colorectal cancer. Emslie et al. took a qualitative approach obtaining extended interviews with each member of the couples they studied and did content analysis to identify themes related to how men and women dealt with the experience of support. The authors noted that caregiving included "caring for," by which they meant practical, work-like activities, such as preparing and serving meals, providing transport, etc. It included "caring about" as well: providing emotional support, listening, sharing feelings, and generally helping to maintain each other's psychological well-being. This part of care was called emotional labor, noting that "management of emotions (one's own and other people's) is hard, skilled work."

While the caregiver provided emotional support as well as practical support, their partners who had cancer also provided emotional support and concern for their spouses who had to cope with the fears and stresses associated with caregiving and the illness of someone they cared for. Mutual support and reciprocity was a key feature of their relationship as judged from their narrative reports.

Marks et al. (2008) focused their attention on transition to the caregiver role, adult children providing care for a parent. The authors drew on the life course perspective and the notion of linked lives. They noted that developmental trajectories of family members are interdependent, that transitions for one family member have consequences for other family members. For elderly parents, the transition may involve health problems and/or aging and transition to frailty and needing assistance while their sons or daughters transitioned to caregiver roles.

Over the life course, the early course of relationships shapes the nature of relationships later in life. For example, Colletti (1997) studied women who became caregivers for their mothers. She noted that the mother—daughter relationships included potential stressors for caregivers. The purpose of Colletti's research was to examine whether the previous quality of the mother-daughter relationship had an effect on burden once the daughters became primary caregivers for their elderly mothers with dementia. Results showed that the history of the relationship mattered. Women who reported better past relationships with their mothers experienced significantly less burden in caregiving compared to women who reported less positive relationship history. This research also demonstrates the point about linked lives. The life course pattern of these women's relationships, both the daughters and mothers, shaped their interaction when they reached the stage where the mothers transitioned to a dependency role and the daughters transitioned to the caregiver role (Ireland and Packenham 2010).

Thomas (2011) directed attention to the interdependence of lives in shared relationships and noted links between social relations and health. Social relations can encourage health promoting behaviors and discourage health risk behaviors and can buffer stressful conditions and events. Thomas applied the life course perspective to study, "how changes in social engagement, over time, may influence … trajectories of physical and cognitive limitations" of older adults. She had data on persons age 60 or older who participated in the American's Changing Lives panel study that began in 1986 and re-interviewed participants in 1989, 1994, and 2002. Participants were mainly women (67.1 %) and most were white (68.5 %).

Thomas specifically made a distinction between formal roles and other kinds of social engagements since older folk often lose formal roles like the worker role. It was noted that older adults can still have continuity in social relationships and social activities that link their lives to others and remain socially integrated despite role changes. So, social engagement here referred to the extent of involvement in social activities like talking to friends and neighbors, visiting relatives, friends, and neighbors, attending community or religious gatherings, and doing volunteer work. Results of this research, consistent with Thomas' hypothesis, were that "social attachment through social engagement has potentially protective effects on cognitive and physical limitations" (p. 439).

Sims-Gould et al. (2008) also noted the nature of linked lives when they studied the effect of crises in caregiving when caregivers were employed persons providing care for older relatives. Data from three waves of interviews (1991 to 1995) indicated that about half (47 %) of caregivers in the study experienced at least one crisis in the 6 months prior to the study. Most of these crises were health related episodes of the care receiver though some crises included financial or family events in the lives of the caregiver or care receiver.

Those who experienced crises reported significantly more changes in their job responsibilities, absenteeism, changes in their participation in non-job activities such as community work and leisure activities and even disruption of sleep, rest, and socializing. As Sims-Gould et al. pointed out, lives are linked over the life course. A change in the life of one family member can result in crises and change for other members, such as ones providing care. In response to crises, "events… above and beyond their caregiving responsibilities," caregivers made adaptations in their work and personal lives to see that the needs of their older relative were met (p. 135). Throughout the life course, lives are linked in a variety of relationships. Family relationships are an important example. Relationships grow and change. Normative demands include emotional bonds of affection and caring concern as well as reciprocal responsibilities. As these develop over the life course, these normative bonds form the basis for caregiving.

The life course trajectory of relationships within a family and the life stage of both caregiver and care recipient form the context of caregiving. Motivation of the caregiver and the ability of the caregiver and care receiver to negotiate this new phase of their relationship are involved. Also, resources of time, money, and energy differ at various life stages as well.

Consider a not uncommon situation where adults in middle adulthood are faced with the disability of a parent in the later adulthood stage. The typical themes of middle adulthood—the developmental tasks—are management of a household, childrearing, managing one's career. Middle adulthood is also a time when many adults are active in their communities. Taking on the caregiver role in middle adulthood may require having to decide about redirecting funds that were earmarked for children's education and/or their own retirement. Caregiving may create role conflicts among career, parenting, marital, community, and caregiving roles.

Pearlin et al. (2001) studied the effect of persons adding the caregiver role to their existing role-set. Their sample was made up of adults whose mother or father was the spousal caregiver to the other, non-institutionalized parent with Alzheimer's disease. The authors noted that normative emotional bonds exist. Family members establish attachments across generations that develop over the life course. These attachments include devotion and concern for the well-being of family members. Affection and concern for parents and grandparents can develop over the life course that can also create a sense of responsibility to provide assistance and care if/when they become disabled. The norms of family bonds led these researchers to expect that the extent of the impaired parent's needs and health problems of the spousal caregiver would influence the extent of their adult children's involvement in the caregiving. They also expected the quality of the adult children's relationship with their parents to influence their participation. However, these expected outcomes were not supported by the data. Role conflicts, commitment to employment, and financial concerns were found to be significantly related to the extent of caregiving assistance these adult children were able to provide. These results demonstrated how the life course stages were involved in the course of caregiving.

The phrase, "The Sandwich Generation" has been applied to the situation where some family members have responsibilities for both younger and older family members. The sandwich idea refers to being at a life stage where one is pressed between those above—an older generation—and those below—a younger generation. The phrase "calls attention to the conflicts and dilemmas that adult children or grandchildren experience in providing care to an impaired relative while at the same time having obligations to other activities and relationships, especially their own children" (Pearlin et al. 2001).

Marks et al. (2008) studied the transition to caregiving. They asserted that the life course context mediated the effects of caregiving on caregiver's well-being and health as both caregiver and care receiver take on new roles and the trajectory of their relationship makes a transition. The transition to the caregiver role is also conditioned upon the role set of the caregiver, whether this role is taken on with or without other major roles like spouse, parent, and worker. The health effects of taking on the caregiver role are also likely to be related to the role set.

Marks et al. also specified other important factors that establish the context of caregiving and affect the health effects of the transition, the increased burden and psychological distress. These include caregiver's age, gender, and education, race/

ethnicity and the cultural context, the relationship history of caregiver and care receiver, and caregiver's appraisal or meaning they attach to the situation. Also included are opportunities and constraints of social location and household income both current and over the life course.

Data for their study came from the National Survey of Families and Households, a nationally representative sample of adults. Two sets of personal interviews were conducted, the first taken in 1987 and 1988, the second between 1992 and 1994. From the original sample, respondents who were between age 25 and 65, who were not caregiving, who had only one living parent at the time of the first interview, and who were caregiving for a parent out of their household at the time of the second interview were selected for this analysis. The analysis focused on four outcome measures: depressive symptoms, happiness, self-esteem and sense of mastery, and self ratings of health.

Research results, as reported by Marks et al. revealed that those sons and daughters who made the transition to caregiving between the two interviews had a greater increase in depressive symptoms compared to those who did not begin to provide care (p. 377). The analysis also showed gender effects; employed women engaged in caregiving a parent had higher depressive symptoms and less psychological wellness than men who were filial caregivers. Women caregivers with below median income had a lower sense of personal mastery compared to their male counterparts. However filial care and being unmarried added more to men's depressive symptoms than to women's and a lower sense of filial obligation upon becoming a caregiver decreased men's happiness more than women's.

Marks et al. also tested hypotheses about the life course relationship quality with parent prior to the start of caregiving. Generally, the hypothesis states that the quality of health and well-being outcomes is directly related to the quality of the relationship; poor relationship, poor outcomes. They claimed only partial support for this hypothesis. Women who had poorer relationships with their parents had greater declines in self-esteem compared to women who had more positive relationships. There was also a trend that daughters with poor relationships had greater declines in physical health while caregiving. But contrary to expectations, poor relationship history seemed to buffer the affect of caregiving on depressive symptoms among women. The hypothesis seemed to work better with men. Those men who had poor relationships experienced poorer psychological outcomes from caregiving.

Some hypotheses about social position were also tested. Not surprisingly low income made a difference; daughters with low income reported poorer health than higher income caregiving daughters. But lower income and lower levels of education was sometimes associated with better well-being than those with more advantages. Lower income caregiving women had significantly less increase in depressive symptoms and lower levels of hostility (a measure of psychological well-being) then those with higher income. Low income caregiving men reported higher levels of mastery and greater increases in happiness than their higher income counterparts.

Employment affected women more than men. Employed daughter caregivers had more hostility, less mastery, and less psychological well-being than those not employed but no such difference was found among the men who became caregivers. The combination of caregiver role and worker role led to increased role conflict and stress on the women. The parent role also made some differences. Parenting made no difference for daughter caregivers, but being a parent provided a benefit to men's psychological wellness compared to those male caregivers who were not parents of young children.

Pavalko and Woodbury (2000) also studied effects of the transition to caregiving. Where Marks et al. studied out-of-home caregivers, Pavalko and Woodbury studied the transition to in-home caregiving. Their data was drawn from two waves of interviews (1987 and 1989) of the National Longitudinal Survey of Mature Women, a nationally representative sample of women which started in 1967 when the women were between 30 and 44 years of age. In 1987 the women were between 50 and 65. The analysis sample included 2,929 women, 2,622 who were not involved in caregiving in 1987. Ninety-four women began caregiving between 1987 and 1989, 86 were already involved in long term caregiving, and 127 stopped caregiving during the period of study. Outcomes studied included extent of physical health limitations and psychological distress.

Results showed relationships between caregiving and health measures in 1989. The women who started caregiving after 1987 showed an increase in physical limitations. Those who were already caregivers in 1987 reported significantly more emotional health problems and physical limitations compared to non-caregivers. Those who stopped caregiving reported particularly high levels of physical limitations which may have had something to do with their having stopped in-home caregiving. Women who stopped continued to experience health declines. Compared to the non-caregivers, those who started caregiving had increased levels of distress, but the long-term caregivers, including those who stopped, reported the highest levels of emotional distress, suggesting an accumulation of distress over time.

Health changes showed moderate increases in physical limitations fairly soon after starting caregiving, but the rate of change seemed to level off indicating adaptation. The most significant increases in physical limitations were of the women who stopped caregiving and persisted at least two years after care stopped suggesting slow recovery.

Employment did not seem to affect these women's entry into caregiving. But those already caregiving in 1987 were less likely to be employed at that time. Employment appeared to have a strong effect on increases in women's physical limitations. On the other hand, health appeared to be a factor in women's starting employment. Those with the lowest level of physical limitation were more likely to start employment. While physical health was found to be related, emotional health was unrelated to employment or change in employment status.

Health effects of caregiving differed by employment status. For those who started caregiving, women who were not employed had larger increases in physical health limitations. Women who were long term caregivers showed less health limitation, their leveling off indicated adaptation following an initial decline in health. Results showed that employment may be a buffer against health decline for women during the early stages of caregiving but women's involvement in multiple roles affected their health and well-being.

3.1 Caregiving and the Life Course

Caregiving may occur at any stage in the life course. For example, children or adolescents may have to participate in the care of a parent or grandparent. Young adult parents may have a child with a developmental disability or a serious mental illness. The costs of care and the process of dealing with service systems may affect parent's careers, health, and other aspects of adult development. Seltzer et al. (2001) conducted a longitudinal study in which they "[examined] the extent to which having a child with either a developmental disability or a serious mental health problem can alter the parents' life course and affect their well being at two points in adulthood: when the parents [were] in their mid-30s [1975/1977] and about 15 years later, when they [were] in their early 50s [1992/1994]" (p. 265).

Seltzer et al. called attention to a timing difference for parents since developmental disabilities are usually diagnosed early in the child's life or even at birth, while mental illness may not emerge until later in the child's adolescence or early adulthood. The onset of caregiving would therefore occur at different stages in the parent's life course—"early adulthood for parents of children with developmental disabilities, and mid-life for parents of persons with severe mental health problems" (p. 266).

Consistent with the life course perspective, Seltzer et al. noted recent influences of the larger social context and historical developments. Prior to the 1990s, mental health professionals and society at large were likely to identify parenting as the cause of the child's mental illness, while parents of children with developmental disabilities were less stigmatized. Also, recent legislation and community-based services and school-based services have come to the aid of children with developmental disabilities and their families. Results of this study showed that parents of persons with a developmental disability had lower rates of employment and lower rates of social participation. These parents had made an adaptation of their employment by working fewer hours which continued into their midlife stage.

Caregiving itself has a life course that includes the stage of the actual onset of caregiving responsibilities. Other stages may be prompted by changes in the health trajectory of care receiver or caregiver. It may include a stage of increasing need for in-home professional services. Medical needs often result in hospital care with regular visits to the hospital by the caregiver. Another stage may be return home and a convalescence period. Eventually caregivers and care receiver may be faced with the difficult decision about out-of-home placement in a nursing home or assisted living facility.

And, for many persons caregiving ends. Aneshensel et al. (2004) conducted a panel study of caregivers that involved six face-to-face interviews over 6 years. The respondents were spouses or adult children, primary caregivers for noninstitutionalized persons suffering from dementia. The authors noted the onset of caregiving can be stressful because of the changes affecting a loved one who can no longer care for themselves. The transition introduces a new life course trajectory that may include costs and losses as well as role conflicts. The death of the care recipient may end caregiving but may have a continuing effect because of bereavement and the role adaptations the caregiver had made when taking on the caregiving role.

Aneshensel et al. also emphasized that lives are linked and interdependent. The links existed before the onset of caregiving—the bonds of marriage or the bond between child and parent. The involvement in caregiving is a major behavioral commitment affecting many aspects of the caregiver's life. The death of the family member cared for is a stressful life event which occurs in the context of the stressful situation of caregiving that includes giving care to a loved one with a degenerative and fatal condition. Bereavement follows the death with its affect on the caregiver's well-being and emotional distress. Results of the study showed that various trajectories of bereavement and symptoms of distress followed the death of the family member who had been cared for.

Orzeck and Silverman (2008) asserted that the post-caregiving stage is a part of the caregiving life course that has received little attention from professional service providers. They noted that caregiving includes various stages like the onset but may also include out-of-home placements, hospital visits, etc. They expressed their view that the post-caregiving stage should be recognized by practice. Caregivers have ongoing needs long after the death of the one cared for. These caregivers must deal with transitions and losses during the post caregiving stage. They had to deal with a loss when they recognized the changes in their family member that occasioned the need for caregiving. Now, they must deal with the loss of their loved one, but they may have also had losses of career and social contacts and activities in adapting to caregiving and now must face these losses as well. The commitment to caregiving, with attendant lifestyle adjustments, may have required the post-caregiving person to need to address identity issues. Like many other life events, the transition to the post-caregiving stage includes stress and a need for adaptation.

3.2 Summary

Caregiving involves a relationship between a person who has become disabled and a person or persons who provide care. The Life Course Perspective offers a framework for situating and understanding the many variations in caregiving. The perspective recognizes the various life stages, each with specific needs and associated roles. Caregiving will be significantly affected depending on the life stage of both caregiver and care receiver.

Our previous comment about the Sandwich Generation is an example. Adults who have minor children who are caring for an elderly parent or grandparent have competing demands for their time and finances. Funds that they may need to provide for their children's education may also be needed in the care of their parent. Their careers and other activities such as community involvements or recreation may also compete. These caregiving adults are in a life stage where childrearing and career and community involvements are significant.

Older adults in a post-parental stage may also become caregivers for a disabled parent, relative, or friend. Such adults, perhaps in their 60s, may be faced with decisions about devoting funds to their caregiving that perhaps they were counting on for their own retirement.

The life stage of the onset of caregiving sets the resources and competing demands that the caregiver must adapt to. The life stage of the onset of disability requiring caregiving is another important variable. Young adults or even midlife adults who become disabled and recipients of care may find becoming dependent inconsistent with their self image. They may have to deal with their inability to enact valued family and other roles. Their previous relationship with the person or persons that become their caregivers take on new dimensions.

Another example of this is when a child of young parents has a developmental disability. The parents are at a life stage at the beginnings of their careers and financial resources may be limited. The child's development through the typical life stages may not occur as expected causing various consequences for the parents and for their other children. Again, the life course stage of both caregiver and care recipient establishes the basis on which caregiving develops.

The life course perspective also emphasizes the impact of the socio-cultural context. Caregiving can be affected by social arrangements that exist in a particular historical era. These social arrangements include scientific developments affecting disability, care, health, and medical procedures. They also include economic conditions that may affect resources available in the provision of care. Also important are legislation and governmental programs and policies that may include things like health insurance, social services, home health assistance, family leave policies, availability of assistive technologies, special education programs, and so on. Public attitudes and media attention that might influence public attitudes are also aspects of social arrangements that may shift over time and affect policies and programs as well as attitudes toward persons with disabilities.

Thus, to conclude, we agree with Hareven (2001) who asserted the value of the life course perspective for understanding caregiving. She noted that patterns of giving support and care as well as expectations of receiving care emerge out of ongoing interaction and relationships between parents and children or among extended family members or fictive kin that are formed and develop over time. In addition, problems and needs develop, accumulate and are shaped over the life course as well. Hareven also noted cohort differences in expectations. Hareven and Adams (1982) found that pre-migration history of ethnic groups affected expectations of support in later life. For older cohorts, support from family members was the expectation while younger cohorts relied on social/governmental programs (Hareven 2001). Earlier life events, as influenced by historical circumstances, also affects the resources—time, money, information, and social networks—available for caregiving. Hareven concluded that to understand the complexities of expectations and patterns of support in later life, we must try to understand "both the social milieu at the time at which members of a cohort reach that age and their cumulative experiences as shaped by historical events".

3.3 Questions for Discussion

1. What is the "convoy model" and its relevance to caregiving?
2. Explain "the Sandwich Generation" and its relevance to caregiving.
3. Explain "caregiving itself has a life course."
4. What is the "post-caregiving" stage?
5. Discuss how life course conditions promote a person's sense of mastery.

References

Aneshensel, C. S., Botticello, A. I., & Yamamoto-Mitani, N. (2004). When caregiving ends. *Journal of Health and Social Behavior, 45,* 422–440.

Antonucci, T. C., Birdett, K. S., Sherman, C. W., & Trinh, S. (2011). Stability and change in the intergenerational family: A convoy approach. *Aging and Society, 31,* 1084–1106.

Bruhn, J. G. (2011). *The sociology of community connections* (2nd ed.). New York: Springer.

Coletti, K. (1997). Adult daughters caring for their elderly mothers with dementia: Impact of prior relationship on caregiver burden. (Unpublished doctoral dissertation: Adelphi University, Garden City, New York).

Crosnoe, R. (2000). Friendships in childhood and adolescence: The life course and new directions. *Social Psychology Quarterly, 63,* 377–391.

Crosnoe, R., & Elder Jr., G. H. (2002). Successful adaptation in the later years: A life course approach to aging. *Social Psychology Quarterly, 65,* 309–328.

Elder Jr., G. H. (1974). *Children of the depression.* Chicago: University of Chicago Press.

Elder Jr., G. H. (1975). Age differentiation and the life course. *Annual Review of Sociology, 1,* 165–190.

Emslie, C., Browne, S., MacLeod, U., Rozmovits, L., Mitchell, E., & Ziebland, S. (2009). "Getting through" not "going under": A qualitative study of gender and spousal support after diagnosis with colorectal cancer. *Social Science and Medicine, 68,* 1169–1175.

George, L. (1993). Sociological perspectives on life transitions. *Annual Review of Sociology, 19,* 353–373.

Hareven, T. K., & Adams, K. J. (1982). (Eds.) Aging and life course transitions: An introductory perspective. New York: Guilford Press.

Hareven, T. K. (2001). Historical perspectives on aging and family relations. In R. H. Binstock & L. K. George (Eds.), *Handbook of aging and the social sciences* (5th ed., pp. 141–159). San Diego: Academic Press.

Hutchinson, E. D. (2008). *Dimensions of human behavior* (3rd ed.). Thousand Oaks: Sage Publications.

Ireland, M. J., & Packenham, K. I. (2010). Youth adjustment to parental illness or disability: The role of illness characteristics, caregiving and attachment. *Psychology and Medicine, 15*(6), 632–645.

Kahn, J. R., & Pearlin, L. I. (2006). Financial strain over the life course and health among older adults. *Journal of Health and Social Behavior, 41,* 17–31.

Marks, N. F., Lambert, J. D., Jun, H., & Song, J. (2008). Psychosocial moderators of the effects of transitioning into filial caregiving on mental and physical health. *Research on Aging, 30*(3), 358–389.

Orzeck, P., & Silverman, M. (2008). Recognizing post-caregiving as part of the caregiving career: Implications for practice. *Journal of Social Work Practice, 22,* 211–220.

Pavalko, K., & Woodbury, S. (2000). Social roles as process: Caregiving careers and women's health. *Journal of Health and Social Behavior, 41,* 91–105.

Pearlin, L. I., Pioli, M. F., & McLaughlin, A. E. (2001). Caregiving by adult children: Role disruption and health. In R. H. Binstock & L. K. George (Eds.), *Handbook of aging and the social sciences* (5th ed., pp. 238–254). San Diego: Academic Press.

Pearlin, L. I., Schieman, S., Fazio, E. M., & Meersman, S. (2005). Stress, health, and the life course: Some conceptual perspectives. *Journal of Health and Social Behavior, 46,* 205–219.

Pearlin, L. I., Nguyen, K. B., Schieman, S., & Milke, M. A. (2007). The life course origins of mastery among older people. *Journal of Health and Social Behavior, 48*(2), 164–179.

Seltzer, M. M., Greenberg, J. S., Floyd, F. J., Pettee, Y., & Hong, J. (2001). Life course impacts of parenting a child with a disability. *American Journal on Mental Retardation, 106,* 265–286.

Sims-Gould, J., Martin-Matthews, A., & Gignac, M. A. M. (2008). Episodic crises in the provision of care to elderly relatives. *Journal of Applied Gerontology, 27,* 123–140.

Thoits, P. A. (2006). Personal agency in the stress process. *Journal of Health and Social Behavior, 47,* 309–323.

Thomas, P. A. (2011). Trajectories of social engagement and limitations in late life. *Journal of Health and Social Behavior, 52*(4), 430–444.

Chapter 4
Caregiving Children with Special Healthcare Needs

4.1 Introduction

Much of what has been written on caregiving and much of public and media attention has concerned eldercare and women aged 50 and older who become caregivers for spouses or aging parents. But, for some families the need for caregiving arises earlier in the life course when faced with children's disabilities and special healthcare needs. Table 4.1 lists some of the conditions that often afflict children and present the need for more than ordinary care. Estimates of the prevalence of children with special healthcare needs range from about 12 to 18 % of children in the United States (Szilagyn 2012; Leiter et al. 2004; Kuo et al. 2011; Karaca-Mandic et al. 2013).

4.2 Estimates of Prevalence of Children with Special Needs

The Maternal and Child Health Bureau (MCHB) defined children with special healthcare needs, "... as those children who have or are at increased risk for a chronic physical, developmental, behavioral, or emotional condition and who also require healthcare related services of a type or amount beyond that required by children generally" (Van Dyck et al. 2004, p. 884). The conditions listed in Table 4.1 do indeed qualify according to this definition.

One purpose of the *National Survey of Children with Special Health Care Needs* is to estimate the prevalence of these children within the population. Households are contacted and the presence of children with special healthcare needs is determined by parents' answers to screening questions: did their child use more medical care, mental health services, or educational services than is usual for most children of the same age? Did the child need prescription medications or therapies and above routine need for, or use of, medical, mental health, or educational services? Was the child limited or prevented in any way in his or her ability to do things that most other children their age can do because of a medical, behavioral, or other health

J. G. Bruhn, H. M. Rebach, *The Sociology of Caregiving*,
Clinical Sociology: Research and Practice, DOI 10.1007/978-94-017-8857-1_4,

Table 4.1 Health conditions considered special healthcare needs

Attention deficit disorder	Depression
Attention deficit hyperactive disorder	Behavioral problems
Autism	Anxiety problem
Asperger's	Autism spectrum disorders (ASD)
Intellectual disability	Developmental delay
Epilepsy	Migraines
Traumatic brain injury	Heart problems
Cystic fibrosis	Blood problems
Cerebral palsy	Muscular dystrophy
Arthritis	Down syndrome
Joint problems	Allergies

condition that is expected to last at least 1 year? The child was considered a child with special healthcare needs if parents answered yes to all these questions.

Van Dyck et al. (2004) reported on the 2001 *National Survey of Children with Special Health Care Needs* conducted jointly by the Maternal and Child Health Bureau and the Center for Health Statistics. The purpose of the survey was to determine the prevalence of and to identify special healthcare needs children, to obtain information on their functional status and services use and to gain information on families' experiences with the healthcare system. The survey was administered to a nationally representative sample of U.S. households, screened for the presence of children who met the MCHB definition. The analysis sample included 38,866 respondents.

The 2001 survey led to an estimate of 12.8 % or an estimated 9.3 million children in the United States, younger than 18 who met the MCHB definition. Boys were reported to be 50 % more likely to be children with special healthcare needs. Also older children were twice as likely to meet the criteria compared to children less than age six. Also, children of families living with incomes below the federal poverty level were significantly more likely to meet the criteria as children with special healthcare needs.

The 2005 survey estimated that 13.9 % or about 10.2 million U.S. children were children with special healthcare needs. The 2009–2010 survey estimated 15.1 % or about 11.2 million U.S. children have special healthcare needs. And, 23.0 % of U.S. households with children have at least one such child. In the 2009–2010 data, 17.4 % of boys compared to 12.7 % of girls were children with special needs. School age children were more likely to be special needs children compared to preschoolers. The rates by age were 18 % ages 6–11, 18 % ages 12–17, compared to 9.3 % ages 0–5. Prevalence also varies somewhat by income and by race/ethnicity (U.S. Department of Health and Human Services Administration, & Maternal and Child Health Bureau 2013).

4.3 Caregiving Concerns

The tasks, concerns, and attention of caregivers are centered on and absorbed by making sure that their child gets the medical, healthcare, and support services the child needs. This includes early identification and early intervention, having a regular physician, having referrals for specialist treatments when necessary, having prescription medications as necessary, and having assistance arranging for and coordinating care. Sometimes the child might need specialized care in addition to medical treatments, perhaps speech therapy or physical therapy or occupational therapy or psychotherapy and educational services may be needed. Caregivers who have assistance with referrals and with arranging and coordinating care find the burden reduced and the child gets better care.

Van Dyck et al. (2004) assessed families' use and needs for medical and support services, satisfaction with their child's care, and the impact of the child's condition on the family. They reported disparities in access to medical care. Families from racial and ethnic minorities, families with lower incomes, families without full health insurance coverage, and families where the identified child was usually affected by their condition were more likely to have problems of access to care, unmet needs, and difficulty getting referrals for specialty care. Families whose child was most severely affected by their condition were significantly more likely to report unmet needs for healthcare services and support services and difficulty getting referrals. Families without health insurance were also at high risk of having access problems.

The impact of the child's condition on the family was also assessed. Financial problems resulting from the child's condition were the ones most commonly mentioned, especially by families living close to, at, or below the federal poverty level and families without full health insurance coverage. Another frequently mentioned impact was the effect of caregiving on employment. About a third of respondents reported at least one family member had to reduce or cease their employment because of their child's condition. Families with a severely affected child reported the greatest impact on finances, employment, and time spent each day providing care.

Leiter et al. (2004) provided some description of caregiving children with special healthcare needs. They explored questions about mothers as caregivers of children with special healthcare needs who were also employed. They noted that such caregiving can be time consuming and may involve a variety of atypical activities usually performed by healthcare professionals. Providing home-based therapies, coordination of medical care and advocacy may be among caregiving activities required. They characterized these mothers as "a reserve army of nurses" (p. 382). And the more extensive the disability and the more limitations the child has, the greater the time demands for parents providing care.

Maternal employment often has to be taken into consideration as well, given the financial needs. Leiter et al. (2004) studied the extent that these mothers provided in-home healthcare, the extent that they altered their employment status because of their child's special needs, and effects of caregiving on employment. Data for their study came from the *Family Partners Project,* a project of a national advocacy organization of families of children with special healthcare needs. Respondents had to be parents or grandparents of a child younger than 18 who met the criteria as a child with special healthcare needs. The nationally representative analysis sample included 1,954 caregivers across the U.S.

The children in the sample, average age nine, had a wide range of conditions of special needs. About half of the mothers were home full-time, the rest were divided between full and part-time employment. About a fourth of the mothers had college degrees, 41 % had some college and 32 % had a high school education or less. Incomes ranged from $ 10,000–70,000 with a mean of $ 34,000. Three-fourths of the sample were two-parent families. Eighteen percent of respondents reported they spent 20 h or more in home healthcare per week. On average mothers who reported more caregiving time had children in poor or fair health, children whose conditions were severe or were in unstable condition. Forty-six percent of the children in the sample were technology dependent, that is, their treatment and maintenance required medical devices, and 62 % received some professional home healthcare. Mothers who provided extensive in-home healthcare had lower odds of full-time employment compared to mothers who did not provide such direct care.

More than half of the mothers reported an effect on employment. Of the 984 employed mothers in the sample, 56 % reported they had cut down on their hours at their places of employment. And, on average, children whose mothers had reduced hours of employment had moderate to severe conditions, unstable conditions and 19 % were technology dependent. The majority of the mothers in this sample (65 %) became employed part-time, though mothers who continued full-time still reported reduced hours of paid employment. Those mothers who were at home full-time, 56 % reported quitting because of their child's health needs.

Rupp and Ressler (2009) also provided some descriptions of caregiving for children with disabilities who were also SSI recipients. Data came from *The National Survey of SSI Children and Families,* a nationally representative survey of parents of children who are SSI recipients. The analysis sample included 3,041 respondents; about two thirds of the children involved (2,025) lived in single mother families, the remainder (1,016) lived in two-parent families. Comparison of the distributions of child characteristics like general health status, type and severity of disability and limitations and indicators of healthcare utilization by children with single or two-parent families showed mostly similarities.

One key part of the analysis was the parent inputs that form the context of caregiving. About a third of all the parents had less education than a high school completion and 22.4 % of single mothers, 17.2 % of married mothers, and 15.1 % of married fathers had a disability or significant health condition. These characteristics can be limitations on caregiving. The pattern of labor force participation, paid employment outside the home, showed 43.9 % of single mothers were employed, about two-thirds of whom were employed full time, and 34 % of married mothers were employed also about two thirds full-time, and 66 % of married fathers were employed, almost 90 % of them employed full-time.

There were significant differences in average income. These results indicate that children living in two-parent families have the potential of more parental time available for caregiving and more money available for the purchase of services. However, be reminded that this research was based on children receiving SSI which is a means tested program. Eligibility is based on parents' income so all incomes among these respondents are lower than average. Single mothers were twice as likely to have incomes below the poverty threshold; 38.7 % of single mother families compared to 19.2 % of two-parent families. In addition about half, 50.4 % of two-parent and 45.8 % of single mothers had "near poor" incomes (below 200 % of poverty threshold).

With regard to caregiving, results showed 34.5 % of children of single mothers, 44.7 % of children in two-parent families receive home healthcare, care specifically related to their condition and health needs, from family members. Specifically, 36.3 % of single mothers and 46.2 % of married mothers provided home healthcare and 29.6 % of married fathers also provided home healthcare. Rupp and Ressler interpreted their results as showing that a substantial portion of the children do not receive any tangible family caregiving related to their healthcare needs. Note also that married mothers are likely to provide more care than single mothers. Among those who reported hours, about one-third of mothers—single or married—reported almost the equivalent of a full-time job. Caring for a disabled child with special healthcare needs is time consuming. Paid care, probably because of the expense, was relatively rare. Overall results showed that children living with two parents were more likely to receive care. With two adults in the household there is more parent time available.

Patterns of care for a disabled child during the work hours of the day can be problematic. Most daycare was provided by relatives. Twenty-three percent of single mothers, 16.5 % of two-parent families had unrelated persons—babysitters—or used organized child care facilities. Almost one-third of children living with single mothers received paid-for care.

More generally, it would seem that caregiving children with special healthcare needs frequently becomes a family affair. Respondents indicated family members in addition to parents provided healthcare. Rupp and Ressler reported a significant positive correlation between the severity of the child's condition and the percent of respondents who reported care hours by family members, though this is affected by the nature of the child's condition.

Children with a physical disability were more likely to receive more hours of caregiving than children whose disability was mental or behavioral. Similarly children with limitations on three or more ADLs, and children who were perceived to be affected a great deal by their condition were more likely to get more caregiving time. Children perceived to be "in poor health" were significantly less likely to receive caregiving than similar children not perceived to be in poor health. Family characteristics enter in. The odds of family caregiving increase significantly for children with at least one parent with an education beyond high school compared to parents who did not graduate high school. Having a two-parent family increases the odds of family caregiving by about 50 %. Having another child in the home under 5 years old or another disabled person reduced the odds of receiving caregiving (Rupp and Ressler 2009, p. 167).

The employee role and the mother/caregiver role interact on many levels. Warfield (2001) suggested that characteristics of the parenting role predict well-being on the job and characteristics of the job predict parenting well-being for the mother of children with disabilities. And for both, family characteristics including income, family structure, and family size sets the context. Warfield sampled mothers from *The Early Intervention Collaborative Study,* a longitudinal study of young children with disabilities. Families were recruited for this study when they enrolled in early intervention programs in Massachusetts and New Hampshire. The analysis sample included 122 mothers of children with special healthcare needs who were interviewed within 1 month of each child's fifth birthday.

No significant differences were found between mothers employed full-time and mothers employed part-time or not employed on parenting demands, child's cognitive performance, family support, or parenting stress. Parenting stress was related to parenting demands which was a measure that included the extent of child behavior problems and the difficulty of caregiving tasks. Parenting stress was also related to less family support. Work interest, the extent to which respondents found their jobs interesting, and less work intensity, an indication of the job's demands, were significantly related to lower parenting stress. Greater parenting demands and greater work intensity was significantly related to days missed from the job. Greater work intensity reduced work quality on the job. Work interest moderated the negative influence of parenting demands on stress when parenting demands were low, but high levels of parenting demands were associated with high stress levels despite the level of work interest. Greater parenting demands were also found associated with increased absence from the job.

Information, including information about available intervention strategies was a need expressed by parents with disabilities in a recent survey (Porterfield and McBride 2007). Even if the family has health insurance coverage for specialty care, services use is unlikely unless the parent seeks treatment. Porterfield and McBride examined the association between family poverty, caregivers' education, health insurance coverage, and perceived need for specialized healthcare and use of three types of specialty health services, specialist physicians, developmental therapies, and prescription medication among children with special care needs. They also examined caregivers' reported reasons why some service requests were not met.

Porterfield and McBride used data from the 2001 *National Survey of Children with Special Health Care Needs.* Thirty-seven percent of respondents had incomes below 200 % of the poverty threshold, 43.5 % had at least a high school education. Seventy percent of children were privately insured, 11 % were uninsured for at least 1 month. The most common healthcare need identified was prescription medications. Over half reported need for specialist physician services and many reported need for other kinds of therapy. Parents whose children had activity limitations were significantly more likely to express need for specialist physician services and therapy services. Health insurance played a major role in gaining access to healthcare services. The most common reason children did not receive services was they cost too much.

Access appeared to be mainly influenced by income and the educational status of parents as well as the severity and nature of the child's special needs. Predictably, less educated parents are also likely to be lower income parents. But less educated and lower income parents had a lower perceived need for specialized services. They were likely to report severe functional limitations of their child, but low parent income, lack of insurance, and lower parent education may mean that some children with special needs do not receive services.

4.4 Finances of Caregiving Special Needs Children

The key issue for families with children with special healthcare needs is meeting the child's healthcare needs. At present, in the United States, there is also a financial issue. Karaca-Mandic et al. (2013, p. 1054) reported that children with special healthcare needs accounted for 47.6 % of all children's healthcare expenditures in 2008. They also noted a general decline in healthcare spending in the U.S. related to decreased household income and savings and an increased risk of loss of job and of health insurance, all related to the recession of 2008–2010. They raised the question of whether the recession affected children with special healthcare needs. Data for the study by Karaca-Mandic et al. (2013) came from the *Medical Expenditure Panel Survey, 2001–2009* (MEPS), a nationally representative sample that includes data on healthcare access and use and related information. The results showed that out of pocket spending for typically developing children increased gradually before and during the recession, but out of pocket spending for children with special healthcare needs was much higher. It increased before the recession but actually decreased during the recession, 2007–2009 (p. 1057). It suggests that some special needs children's needs for services were not met.

The national economy is one factor affecting services sought by caregivers of children with special needs. The economy of their state of residence is another factor. Parish et al. (2012) raised questions about state-level income inequality and burden for families with children with special healthcare needs. They noted that, compared to other children, the children with special healthcare needs have increased need for health and specialty care; because of chronic physical, mental, developmental, or behavioral conditions they need increased physician visits, emergency department visits, hospitalizations, medications, procedures, equipment, therapies and supportive services, all of it expensive to families and the public health system. Families' out of pocket payments are part of the caregiving burden which varies from state to state.

Using data from the *National Survey of Children with Special Health Care Needs* collected between April, 2005, and February, 2007, and state level data from archival sources including the Census Bureau, Parish et al. (2012) found that state level income inequality was significantly associated with financial and caregiving burdens experienced by families of children with special healthcare needs. Financial burden refers to a significant proportion of household income devoted to out of pocket healthcare expenditures not including the costs of health insurance. Caregiving burden refers to things like not receiving professional help arranging or coordinating care for the child, or a parent or other primary caregiver who had to cease employment. Lower income families living in states with greater income inequality experienced greater burden.

Analysis of the data showed that a 1 % increase in inequality, measured by the Gini index, was associated with 6 % higher odds that a low income family did not get help arranging for or coordinating healthcare for their child with special healthcare needs. And a 1 % increase in income inequality was associated with 3 % higher odds that a parent ceased employment due to the child's healthcare needs. And a 1 % increase in income inequality was associated with 6 % higher odds of having financial burden of $ 250 to 500 (relative to $ 1–250) and 6 % higher odds of financial burden greater than 3 % of income. Overall the data point to the conclusion that caregivers state of residence is related to financial burden. Caregivers living in states with higher income inequality are likely to experience greater financial burden and the likelihood of children's healthcare needs being met are reduced.

Margolis et al. (2011) were also concerned about how state-level factors related to the well-being of children with special healthcare needs. They particularly noted the trend toward increased state and local governments having responsibility for child health policies and practices and they expressed concern that this trend held "...important implications for child health and well-being" (p. 714). Families of children with special healthcare needs could be affected in terms of dollars spent and services provided. As previously noted there is considerable state to state variation in program eligibility. These differences may have to do with states' capacity. Margolis et al. explored, "… the association between state level economic, political, health systems, and Title V capacities and the well-being of [children with special health care needs]" (p. 714). They hypothesized a direct relationship between state capacity and the well-being of these children. Data on the children and their families came from the *National Survey of Children with Special Health Care Needs* and state capacity and Title V data came from various archival sources.

Results showed some significant relationships between measures of state capacity and outcomes important to the children and their caregivers. State economic capacity, indexed by the gross state product, was associated with care coordination, special education, and less likelihood of using Title V services. The Title V, Maternal and Child Health Program, originally part of the Social Security Act of 1935, is a federal—state partnership program covering mothers, children, and youth including children with special healthcare needs and their families. It became part of the Block Grant Program in 1981. The program can help provide funds as the payer of last resort for services for maternal and child health not covered by other programs. (U.S. Department of Health and Human Services Administration, & Maternal and Child Health Bureau 2013)

Margolis et al. (2011) also found that the greater the percent of state domestic product devoted to health, the more likely the children were to have a usual source of care. Families without health insurance were less likely to receive early intervention and care coordination and more likely to report delay in receiving needed care.

Higher Medicaid managed care enrollment in a state was found associated with families less likely to report use of early intervention services. Also the percentage of children enrolled in Medicaid was positively related to the likelihood of receipt of special education and care coordination services. The higher the per capita gross state product, the more likely children with special needs were to receive special education and care coordination services and less use of Title V services. Increase in the percentage of block grant funds to be spent on children with special healthcare needs was related to more families reporting special education enrollment and more families who had heard of Title V.

There is a great range of needs associated with caregiving for disabled children, and it is all expensive. Susan L. Parish has frequently turned her research attention to the caregiving of children with disabilities and special healthcare needs, especially the economics of it. She joined with colleagues to show the financial impact across the life course on parents of children with disabilities. Parish et al. (2004) were concerned about income and assets at midlife for parents of children with developmental disabilities and the employment trajectories of mothers of these children.

Data for this study came from the *Wisconsin Longitudinal Study* that started in 1957 with a one-third sample of Wisconsin high school seniors with data collected in 1957, 1975, and 1992. The analysis sample for the study included 165 parents with a child with a developmental disability and 165 randomly selected parents without children with special needs for a comparison group. The data analysis showed that parents of children with developmental disabilities had significantly lower annual income and significantly lower savings than comparison parents. Average annual income difference between the two groups was about $ 12,000 and savings of families of children with disabilities was an average 27 % below that of the comparison group (Parish et al. 2004, p. 419–420).

In addition to finances, the study was also interested in mothers' employment patterns. Results showed a significant difference between mothers of children with disabilities and comparison mothers in 1974 income; the comparison mothers earned an average twice that of mothers of children with developmental disabilities, but the average incomes of the two groups were much closer and not significantly different in 1991. As reported, comparison mothers were much more likely to be employed in 1974 (64 % of comparison moms vs. 46 % of mothers of children with developmental disabilities) and employed full-time while mothers of children with disabilities were less likely to be employed and employment was more likely to be part-time. By 1992, when the women were about age 53, their children around age 27, over 80 % of both groups were employed, about 45 % full-time, which probably accounted for the similarity of their incomes at that point. Women's employment was also compared when their children were first born, age 8 and at age 16. The two groups of women appeared to have experienced similar trajectories from their child's birth to adolescence. The likelihood of full-time employment increased as their children got older but the percentage of full-time employment increased more slowly for the mothers of children with developmental disabilities who were somewhat more likely to choose part-time employment. The authors' interpretation of the employment pattern was consistent with the view that care needs of a child with developmental disabilities interferes with their mothers' employment trajectories and earnings. The combination of this and elevated costs of caring for a child with disabilities and special healthcare needs results in diminished savings at midlife.

Parish et al. (2010) also studied the costs, burdens, and financial well-being across the life course of families with children with developmental disabilities. They noted that, "these families often experience drastically altered life course trajectories which result from spending decades in the role of active caregivers" (p. 236). These families may experience "late launching," a delay in the time their children leave the parental home for college, the workforce, and for living as independent adults. The process can be different for children with developmental disabilities or other special healthcare needs.

Parish, Rose, and Swain used data from the 2001 and 2004 panels of the Survey of Income and Program Participation (SIPP) to assess the financial well-being of households with a child older than age five with developmental disabilities. Households were compared by age cohort of the head of household. The sample was divided into four cohorts—under age 45, 45 to 54, 55 to 64, and 65 and older. Results showed that younger parents were more likely to be poor using U.S. federal poverty guidelines. The youngest and oldest cohorts had the lowest incomes and the lowest net worth and liquid assets, though by comparison, the oldest group had considerably more assets than the youngest group. The 55 to 64 cohort of parents had the highest net worth, but net worth declined sharply for those facing retirement.

Overall, Parish, Rose, and Swain interpreted their results as "troubling evidence" about the "precarious financial situation of parents caring for their children with developmental disabilities" (p. 241). Income poverty and asset poverty becomes part of the burden of caregiving. A lack of savings and other assets that can be drawn on to respond to crises, as well as for future needs like education and retirement, leave these families financially vulnerable, especially as they age.

Birdsong and Parish (2008) expressed the opinion that passage of the Healthy Families Act would provide some help to parents, especially women, who face the dilemma of needing the employment and the wages but also face needing to care for their child. They noted that most low income workers do not receive sick leave or family leave; when the child at home needs parental attention the parent faces the choice of losing a day's pay from wages that are low to begin with. They assert that the proposed Act would provide leave for workers who need to take care of themselves or family members. Most workers who are allowed paid sick leave are to use it only when the worker him/herself is ill and is not allowed to use it to care for family members.

Most people with disabilities—not only children—live with family caregivers and most received little public assistance. It was therefore asserted that passage of the Healthy Families Act would provide security and financial security to caregivers and care receivers as well. The Act if passed would require paid sick leave for workers who are employed for at least 20 h per week and for companies with 15 or more employees. Employees would be permitted to earn paid sick leave which could also be used to attend to family members. Assigned to committee in March, 2013, the bill was given a 2% chance of being enacted (GovTrack.U.S. 2013).

Bellin et al. (2011) described the family centered care approach (FCC) to caring for children with special healthcare needs. It was described as an approach that simultaneously supports "… the health and psychosocial well-being of the child and attendance to the needs of surrounding family members including siblings" (Bellin et al. 2011, p. 281). It is meant to acknowledge and mobilize the strengths of the family and to empower the family and to be culturally sensitive. It emphasizes partnership and collaboration between professional healthcare providers and parents and includes family decision making on services choices. The level of family participation in care decision making is set at the families desired level. Attention to the needs of each member of the family system is also an important feature.

The research conducted by Bellin et al. was to compare parent perceptions and provider perceptions of the degree to which FCC practices were being carried out. Study participants included parents of children with special needs whose child had received either inpatient or outpatient services at a hospital and a sample of providers of services to children with special healthcare needs. Results showed that professionals and parents generally agreed on their evaluation of FCC practices and the extent of FCC implementation.

Kuo et al. (2011) also studied family centered care to examine outcomes for the children with special healthcare needs. Their study also included family burden such as access needs, financial and caregiver burdens and child health, stability of child's health and healthcare resource use. They noted that the Maternal and Child Health Bureau, in its 2007 agenda for children with special healthcare needs included Family Centered Care as a core aspect of its recommended system of care with a strong partnership between the family and the providers as the foundation, a partnership based on mutual respect, information sharing, and working together. "Health care that is family centered directly responds to family concerns and priorities" (Kuo et al. 2011, p. 795).

The data for this study came from the 2005–2006 version of the *National Survey of Children with Special Health Care Needs*. They found that 65.6 % of respondents reported family centered care. Younger age, female parent, white parent with higher education levels were found to be predisposing characteristics for FCC. Private insurance, higher income, having a usual source of care and having English as the primary language were also associated with having FCC and were called enabling characteristics.

Analysis of outcomes was conducted by matching FCC families and non-FCC families based on propensity characteristics. Compared to non-FCC families, families with family centered care had improved access to health services and reduced financial burden. They also spent fewer hours in direct caregiving. Families with FCC had lower odds of delayed medical care and unmet services needs. They had fewer problems with referrals and received more help with care coordination. Families with family centered care had higher odds of receiving 18 needed services like home healthcare, specialty care, and useful technology. Family centered care was also found positively related to the child's health stability and less severity. And having FCC was associated with increased emergency room use and increased likelihood of physician visits (Kuo et al. 2011, p. 801).

Based on the above, authors concluded that family centered care as a system of care for children with special healthcare needs is associated with less family burden and efficient health care for children with special healthcare needs and may be particularly desirable for those conditions that are especially difficult to get timely care referrals and other services for.

4.5 Summary

Caregiving children with special healthcare needs enters early into the life course of young parents and may deflect their life course trajectory. Caregiving for children with special needs can involve parents taking on caregiving tasks often associated with nurses and other healthcare professionals. And it may also have an adverse effect on family finances and asset accumulation as parents age. For single parents and other low income families the financial burden can be particularly difficult to bear. These families have few places to turn though many could possibly find help from Title V if they only knew of it. As we write, Health Care Reform is not fully rolled out and The Healthy Families Act remains in committee.

Family centered care, a system of care encourage by the Maternal And Child Health Bureau, establishes a collaborative relationship between the parents/caregivers of children with special healthcare needs and has been the object of recent evaluative research. It seems to offer effective and supportive help for those families that have participated. Still, the development of a well-planned, well organized societal program of child health and psychosocial care would be a benefit to the afflicted children and the parents who struggle to meet their child's special needs.

4.6 Questions for Discussion

1. Given the size of the population affected, should there be a planned, organized societal response to the care of children with special healthcare needs, with respect to the financial aspect as well and treatment structures?
2. Think about the cost of public financing of institutional care for children with special healthcare needs. Compared to that, is there an argument for providing assistance for parent/caregivers to maintain caregiving at home?
3. Discuss some of the effects special needs children have on the family unit and adjustments required to meet those needs.
4. Although improvements have been made in healthcare quality and some disparities have been reduced, differences persist in healthcare quality among children from racial and ethnic minority groups. Children in low-income families and uninsured families also experience poorer quality care. Discuss the implications of disparities in special needs populations.
5. Research shows that special needs children respond better to various therapies when their parents participate in burnout prevention activities. Discuss.

References

Bellin, M. H., Osteen, P., Heffernan, C., Levy, J. M., & Snyder-Vogel, M. E. (2011). Parent and health care professional perspectives on family centered care for children with special health care needs: Are we on the same page? *Health and Social Work, 36*(4), 281–290.

Birdsong, S., & Parish, S. L. (2008). The healthy families act: Vital support for families of people with developmental disabilities. *Intellectual and Developmental Disabilities, 46*(4), 319–321.

GovTrack.us (01 September 2013). Healthy families act (2013). http://www.govtrack.us/congress/bill. Accessed: 1 Sept. 2013.

Karaca-Mandic, P., Yoo, S. J., & Sommers, B. D. (2013). Recession led to a decline in out-of-pocket spending for children with special health care needs. *Health Affairs, 32*(6), 1054–1062.

Kuo, D. Z., Bird, T. M., & Tilford, J. M. (2011). Associations of family-centered care with health care outcomes for children with special health care needs. *Maternal and Child Health, 15,* 794–805.

Leiter, V., Krauss, M. W., Anderson, B., & Wells, N. (2004). The consequences of caring. *Journal of Family Issues, 25*(3), 379–403.

Margolis, L. H., Mayer, M., Clark, K. A., & Farel, A. M. (2011). Associations between state economic and health systems capacities and service use by children with special health care needs. *Maternal and Child Health, 15,* 713–721.

Parish, S. L., Seltzer, M. M., Greenberg, J. S., & Floyd, F. (2004). Economic implications of caregiving at midlife: Comparing parents with and without children who have developmental disabilities. *Mental Retardation, 42*(6), 413–426.

Parish, S. L., Rose, R. A., & Swain, J. G. (2010). Financial well being of US parents caring for coresident children and adults with developmental disabilities: An age cohort analysis. *Journal of Intellectual and Developmental Disability, 35*(4), 235–243.

Parish, S. L., Rose, R. A., Dababnah, S., Yoo, J., & Cassiman, S. A. (2012). State-level income inequality and family burden of US families raising children with special health care needs. *Social Science and Medicine, 74,* 399–407.

Porterfield, S. L., & McBride, T. D. (2007). The effect of poverty and caregiver education on perceived need and access to health services among children with special health care needs. *American Journal of Public Health, 97*(2), 323–329.

Rupp, K., & Ressler, S. (2009). Family caregiving and employment among parents of children with disabilities on SSI. *Journal of Vocational Rehabilitation, 30,* 153–175.

Szilagyi, P. G. (2012). Health insurance and children with disabilities. *Future of Children, 22*(1), 123–147.

U.S. Department of Health And Human Services Administration, & Maternal And Child Health Bureau (2013). *The national survey of children with special health care needs chartbook 2009–2010.* Rockville: U.S. Department of Health and Human Services.

Van Dyck, P. C., Kogan, M. D., McPherson, M. G., Weissman, G. R., & Newacheck, P. W. (2004). Prevalence and characteristics of children with special health care needs. *Archives of Pediatric & Adolescent Medicine, 158*(9), 884–890.

Warfield, M. E. (2001). Employment, parenting, and well-being among mothers of children with disabilities. *Mental Retardation, 39,* 297–309.

Chapter 5
Caregiving Adolescents and Young Adults with Disabilities

5.1 Introduction

For most youth, typically developing youth, later adolescence is the life course stage for anticipating and preparing for the transition to independence and an adult identity. The transition to adulthood includes making decisions about leaving the parental home, joining the workforce or entering college, technical training, or other post secondary education or, perhaps, military service. The transition to adulthood also includes decisions about residence and living arrangements and decisions about peer networks, social and sexual relationships. Young adulthood is the stage when most or all of these decisions have been taken, at least tentatively and the young adult embarks on an attempt at an independent life, loosening the bonds of parental supervision and total support.

It is not always smooth and seamless as the above few lines describe it. But, for many young people, years of parental and cultural expectations communicated in a variety of ways and years of anticipatory socialization for adulthood provide strong stimuli for a more or less normative transition. For young people with disabilities and special healthcare needs and their parents adolescence represents what Parish (2006, p. 394) referred to as "a point of major divergence in the life courses of families raising typically developing children and those raising children with disabilities."

The divergence includes what Heller et al. (2007, p. 248) called delay in the launching phase, the fact that grown children with disabilities or special healthcare needs often continue to live at home and continue to need caregiving. Meanwhile, these youth have often aged out of services from their local school system and services for children and the availability of other sources of services for this age group is often not clear.

J. G. Bruhn, H. M. Rebach, *The Sociology of Caregiving*,
Clinical Sociology: Research and Practice, DOI 10.1007/978-94-017-8857-1_5,

5.2 Service Issues

Parish (2006) listened to the voices of the mothers of adolescents with developmental disabilities. She used focus groups of women who were mothers of and lived with children with developmental disabilities aged 13 to 18, clients of the local disability services organization. The focus group material was coded for themes. The themes that represented the mothers' concerns were about service issues, employment issues, care related issues, and maternal responsibility. The theme of services issues included gratitude for the support services they had received which had been very helpful. However the mothers also noted inadequacies in services, agencies unresponsive to families' needs and a decline in the availability of services for adolescents. Mothers of youth with the most severe behavioral or physical impairments had the most difficult time getting support for their children when school was closed.

Services helpful to caregivers in managing family life were: respite care, summer programs and after school programs and training services. School services were judged by this sample to be inadequate including the need for individualized programs for students with disabilities, late or non-existing transition planning—preparation for life when school days were over—and the decline in available services when their children reached adolescence. It was also interesting that "the participants also expressed frustration with the failure of service providers to recognize that their child's needs were lifelong." For typically developing children, healthcare services were usually temporary but this was not the case with children with developmental disabilities. One mother expressed her feelings, "this thing that is so frustrating… is that it doesn't end" (Parish 2006, p. 398).

Work issues were another theme that Parish identified, specifically the conflict between maintaining employment and meeting caregiving responsibilities. Jobs were considered very important for financial as well as emotional reasons and women had curtailed their involvement in order to provide care. Problems included finding reliable, quality care for their adolescent with developmental disabilities and employed mothers reported juggling their own schedules and the schedules of various care providers to make sure adequate care was present.

Jokinen and Brown (2005) used extensive interviews, focus groups, and survey instruments to study quality of life issues of older parents/caregivers of sons and daughters aged 40 and older with intellectual disabilities. Respondents were asked about their family's quality of life and things that enhanced and detracted. They were also asked about the effect of the person with disability. The main findings showed that these older parents had many common thoughts and perceptions. They viewed themselves as "pioneers" helping to develop a system of services for people with disabilities like their adult children. Parents worked together and saw the benefit of association and expressed positive feelings about the experience. It was not uncommon for them to speak positively about their children's accomplishments. In general respondents in this sample described their family quality of life as good or normal. But difficulties were also mentioned.

These parents were concerned about the future. They wanted more information about aging and intellectual disability for themselves and for their sons and daughters. Their specific concerns included health and how changes in health will affect the family members, themselves as well as their adult child. They wanted to know more about long-term living arrangements and the ability of persons with intellectual disabilities to adapt to age related changes. Many thought the services system was complex and found it difficult to know who to speak to about what and that families could get lost in the shuffle. Finally they were concerned that caregiving would extend beyond their lives and may need to involve other family members. Participants felt that their families needed help and advice on this in order to avert crisis.

5.3 Transition to Adulthood

The transition to adulthood for young people with intellectual disabilities raised philosophical questions about autonomy and decision-making. Murphy et al. (2011, p. 61) noted, "the definition and attribution of the category 'adult' is highly consequential and is negotiated and contested in particular social contexts." With regard to transition aged youth with intellectual disabilities, they identified two conflicting discourses. The first asserts their rights, as adults, to autonomy and self determination. The alternative view questioned their right to self determination based on the individual's lack of capacity for independent practical reasoning and parents' responsibility to make judgments on behalf of the young person.

In their research Murphy, Clegg, and Almack interviewed two cohorts of 18 and 19 year olds with intellectual disabilities as they were completing special schools and they continued following these youth through the transition to adult services in England. Twenty-eight young people, 17 males, participated with levels of disability ranging from mild to profound, though most were in the moderate range. They were interviewed individually three times and six times in small group discussions. Parents/caregivers were also interviewed.

Results revealed that the youth themselves may have been interested in changes that were about to take place but authors reported there was no evidence that adult status was salient for the youth in this sample. Professionals were divided with some asserting that individuals with intellectual disability lacked the capacity for deciding their futures, others said they are capable of making choices and decisions and needed to be included in the process of decision-making over their future care.

Parents appeared to be equivocal, some asserting the youths' adulthood but expressing concern for their care, concern for their vulnerability, and their need for constant supervision. Some looked forward to their child leaving home and the increased freedom they would have though they worried about their children's futures. Parents' ambivalence might be understood as not looking forward to lifetime caregiving but cognizant of their responsibility as parents.

Mill et al. (2009) interviewed young adults with intellectual disabilities on issues of transition to adulthood. In particular, they were concerned about how these individuals negotiated autonomy within their families. In addition to their interest in the issue, these authors also felt that it was important for researchers to listen to the perspective of these young people. The study took a life history approach using two waves of data collection. The first wave used semi-structured interviews. The second wave had more focused in-depth interviews. Autonomy in the family for these youth with intellectual disabilities involved what they wanted and the nature of the parental response.

5.4 Negotiating Autonomy

Results brought out three approaches to negotiating autonomy in the family. They were labeled *defiant*, *passive*, and *proactive*. The key characteristic of the defiant pattern was active protests against parental interference and deliberate rejection of parental authority. The exemplar of this approach, a 20 year old young woman, expressed frustration and hostility and feeling "unheard and under valued in her family and excluded from family ventures…." (Mill et al. 2009, p. 197).

Those passive in their approach appeared not to want significant changes and had been allowed some independence within supervised environments. They often had projects or activities they were involved in within the parental home. They were satisfied with their extent of independence and did not actively seek increased autonomy. The proactive approach was used by those who sought more autonomy and received encouragement for this from their parents who let them learn from their mistakes.

Demographic trends affect caregiving. Heller et al. (2007) like others, noted that increased life expectancies have increased the need for family caregivers while lower fertility rates, smaller families, and increases in dual earner families have reduced the pool of persons who might provide care. They also pointed to the increased life expectancy of persons with developmental disabilities. They concluded that the combination of trends results in an extended period of caregiving required for persons with developmental disabilities and a possible shortage of family members to provide care over the long haul.

Heller et al. also noted that persons with developmental disabilities were less likely to become employed. Family caregiving, which could be for life, can affect the family economically and socially and can have an effect on the health of both caregiver(s) and care receiver. Depression, social isolation, and low levels of maternal psychological well-being are outcomes that have been reported.

Eisenhower and Blacher (2006) were concerned about the well-being of mothers of adolescents and young adults with intellectual disabilities. Their research included 226 mothers whose adolescent or young adult child with intellectual disabilities were in the moderate to severe/profound range and lived at home. These participants were all recruited at regional centers in Southern California. Results showed a significant relationship between mother's health and their psychological well-being. Also a higher rate of problem behaviors by the youth with intellectual disabilities predicted poorer maternal well-being. Well-being was better for those employed and well-being was higher for those married and best for those married and employed. Mothers' well-being was also significantly related to their income and education. As income and educational attainments rose, well-being also rose. Mothers who were unemployed and unmarried had markedly poorer well-being than those employed or married or both. Eisenhower and Blacher also reported that the socio-economic benefits of being married and employed "overshadowed other benefits of role occupancy" (Eisenhower and Blacher 2006, p. 913).

Rapanaro et al. (2008, p. 35) noted that the period of transition to adulthood was an especially challenging and stressful time for parents of young people with an intellectual disability. In addition to the daily demands of caregiving in the transition period, the parents face challenges due to lack of post school services, and issues of dependence/independence, behavior problems, concerns about their child's vulnerability and issues of the long range well-being of their child including guardianship in the event their child will outlive them. Given the potential for stress and negative outcomes Rapanaro, Bartu, and Lee chose to explore both positive and negative outcomes reported by these parents/caregivers.

With the assistance of a state disability services agency, parents of individuals with intellectual disability were recruited for participation in this study. One hundred nineteen respondents that had a son or daughter with an intellectual disability who was between ages 16 and 21 and was cared for at home were included in the study; 58.8 % had a child with mild disability, 33.6 % with moderate disability and 7.6 % cared for a child with severe or profound intellectual disability. At least one stressful event in the previous 12 months was reported by 79 % of respondents: behavior of the young adult (38.3 %), service provider issues (22.3 %), health problems (13.8 %), and young adult vulnerability (9.6 %).

Problem behaviors of the young adults involved aggressiveness, inappropriate behaviors, and sexual behaviors, as well as difficulty adapting to post school settings like jobs and sheltered workshops. Difficulties with service providers were accessing services, actions of services staff, and dissatisfaction with services. A common problem mentioned was specifically services for this age group. Parents also identified their own lack of independence, sadness, feelings of resentment, feelings of being cut off from social contacts, feeling captive in the caregiver role, and how it is likely to continue well into their child's adulthood. But some positive outcomes and positive appraisals were reported.

One positive outcome mentioned were parents becoming more assertive and resourceful at solving problems related to their child's care and dealing with services providers. Another was the development of new networks of supports within the community. Others were increasing closeness within the family, learning new coping skills, increasing understanding of problem areas and personal growth of son or daughter. About half (45.7 %) of parents in this sample described benefits emerging from stressful events they experienced in dealing with their intellectually disabled son or daughter in this difficult age group (Rapanaro et al. 2008).

A more general approach to the transitions by youth with intellectual disabilities was taken by Neece et al. (2009). They noted that transition indicators like having a job, hours worked, income and social networks might not be completely appropriate for youth with intellectual disabilities. The index they used was parent satisfaction with their young adult's transition as an indicator of transition success. It was also used to assess the effect of their young adult's transition on the family well-being. The general view was that a successful (or unsuccessful) transition has to do with how well the family is doing.

Data for their study was provided by 128 parents of young adults with severe intellectual disability who were ages 19 to 28 and all had exited the school system.

Participants were recruited with the assistance of the Southern California Regional Center, a state network that maintains a registry of persons with intellectual disabilities. Questionnaires and in-home personal interviews as well as unobtrusive observations were all used to gather data.

Results were that about half (52.3 %) of the sample expressed satisfaction with the transition, 43 % were in the transition dissatisfaction group and 4.7 % were unclassifiable. As for family well-being, 55 % were in the high family well-being group, 33 % in the low family well-being group and 12 % could not be classified. The distinctions between the transition satisfaction group and the dissatisfaction group were related to variables related to the young adult, family variables, and variables concerned with services. Specifically, in the transition satisfaction group:

- The young adult showed fewer mental health problems.
- Parents rated the young adult higher in quality of life.
- There was less negative impact on the family.
- There was a lower rate of maternal depression.
- Less worry about the effects of transition on the family.
- Satisfaction with their level of involvement in transition planning.
- The young adult had paid work experience.
- Young adult in work experience rather than treatment environment.

5.5 Transition Satisfaction

Further analysis showed that parental involvement in transition planning was a particularly strong predictor of transition satisfaction. There were also significant differences in family well-being between the transition satisfaction and the transition dissatisfaction groups. The families in the transition dissatisfaction group were mostly placed in the low family well-being category.

White and Hastings (2004) found high levels of depression and anxiety among parents of adolescents with intellectual disabilities. In their sample, 61 % of parents of youth with intellectual disability scored either borderline or abnormal when assessed for anxiety, 36 % borderline or clinical for depression. White and Hastings noted that psychological outcomes for these parents may be affected by available resources with social support a key resource. The research assessed availability and helpfulness and extent of use of social supports, both informal—family, friends, spouses—and formal—professional services. Support was also assessed for the functions served by the support: practical, like help with caring for the child or household help, and emotional support.

Results supported other studies showing that problem behaviors had a major negative affect on parents' well-being. Features of social support increased parents' well-being. Helpful, practical informal supports improved parents' well-being. Professional supports and services did not appear to improve parental well-being however. These supports seemed to be more associated with the needs of the child.

Maintaining family health is an important issue for caregivers, given the potential for stressors. Serious mental illnesses such as schizophrenia often occur during late adolescence or young adulthood and require considerable care. Families provide a major proportion of the care for these young adults. The research of Doornbos (2002) focused on the health of these families that suddenly had to respond to "the challenges associated with a member's [serious mental illness], the magnitude of the responsibilities taken on by the family caregivers, and the minimal preparation and support provided by mental healthcare professionals has the potential to adversely affect the health of these families" (Doornbos 2002, p. 242). The burden may be particularly intense just following the onset of serious mental disorder as the family struggles to adjust to the reality of a member's illness and episodes of problem behaviors. Stressors that arise may be financial, illness related, or legal, marital, or related to employment or housing. Specific factors studied by Doornbos were the family's perception of the symptoms of mental illness, the time since diagnosis, family stressors and coping and communication from professionals.

Communication with mental health professionals was considered an important factor; caregivers had a high need for information and advice. Educational and psychoeducational interventions helped reduce family burden and improve family function and coping as well as improve caregiver well-being.

Traumatic brain injuries, though very different from the kinds of disabilities we have referred to, also have the prospect of long-term caregiving. Wongvatunyu and Porter (2005) did in-depth interviews with seven mothers caring for young adults who had experienced moderate—to—severe injury. Results focus on what these mothers were trying to do. "Reconnecting my child's brain" was one major activity. Mothers sought to retrain or help reprogram their child's brain to have other areas take over functions lost from injury and they tried to help their child set up reminder systems to compensate for memory problems.

Another caregiving activity was monitoring their child's safety and preventing re-injury. A third was "making our lives as normal as possible." This starts with recovery at home, a familiar environment with special attention and care from their mother. Dealing with the biggest problem and advocating for their child were also key tasks, the biggest problem was the child's disability and advocacy was making sure the youth received the care needed.

5.6 Summary

As several investigators have pointed out, the life course stage associated with the transition to adulthood is an especially difficult time for parents/caregivers and for youth with disabilities or special healthcare needs. For parents it can be a time of anxiety about their son or daughter having a normative life course including independence, careers, and families. And parents face the issue of lifelong caregiving and concerns about who will care for their son or daughter beyond their life span. And there are daily issues of medical and other professional support and the question of the dollar costs, now and in the future. As we write, The Affordable Care Act (Obama care) has just started to come on line and may prove especially helpful for families with young adults with disabilities being cared for at home.

5.7 Questions for Discussion

1. Why is the transition stage difficult for parents? What are social, economic, and personal sources of stress that make the period difficult?
2. Why is the transition stage a special challenge for persons with disabilities or special healthcare needs?
3. Take the role of a consultant to families with a young adult with disabilities. What are sources of support for the family? For the young adult with disabilities? Find out, for your area. There is likely to be wide state-to-state variability.
4. Explain the major steps in negotiating autonomy for a family member with disabilities.
5. Discuss the effects of long-term or life-long caregiving on the family system.

References

Doornbos, M. M. (2002). Predicting family health in families of young adults with severe mental illness. *Journal of Family Nursing, 8*(3), 241–263.

Eisenhower, A., & Blacher, J. (2006). Mothers of young adults with intellectual disability: Multiple roles, ethnicity, and well-being. *Journal of Intellectual Disability Research, 50*(12), 905–916.

Heller, T., Caldwell, J., & Factor, A. (2007). Aging family caregivers: Policies and practices. *Mental Retardation and Developmental Disabilities, 13,* 136–142.

Jokinen, N. S., & Brown, R. I. (2005). Family quality of life from the perspective of older parents. *Journal of Intellectual Disability Research, 49*(10), 789–793.

Mill, A., Mayes, R., & McConnell, D. (2009). Negotiating autonomy within the family: The experiences of young adults with intellectual disabilities. *British Journal of Learning Disabilities, 38,* 194–200.

Murphy, E., Clegg, J., & Almack, K. (2011). Constructing adulthood in discussions about the futures of young people with moderate-profound intellectual disabilities. *Journal of Applied Research in Intellectual Disabilities, 24,* 61–73.

Neece, C. L., Kraemer, B. R., & Blacher, J. (2009). Transition satisfaction and family well-being among parents of young adults with severe intellectual disability. *Intellectual and developmental disabilities, 47*(1), 31–43.

Parish, S. L. (2006). Juggling and struggling: A preliminary work-life study of mothers with adolescents who have developmental disabilities. *Mental Retardation, 44*(6), 393–404.

Rapanaro, C., Bartu, A., & Lee, A. H. (2008). Perceived benefits and negative impact of challenges encountered in caring for young adults with intellectual disabilities in the transition to adulthood. *Journal of Applied Research in Intellectual Disabilities, 21,* 34–47.

White, N., & Hastings, R. P. (2004). Social and professional support for parents of adolescents with severe intellectual disabilities. *Journal of Applied Research in Intellectual Disabilities, 17,* 181–190.

Wongvatunyu, S., & Porter, E. J. (2005). Mothers' experience of helping young adults with traumatic brain injury. *Journal of Nursing Scholarship, 37*(1), 48–56.

Chapter 6
Caregiving at Life's Transitions: The Senior Years

6.1 Introduction

Age and time are woven together into the fabric of our society. Life transitions are frequently linked to chronological age—the age to vote or drive a car, or associated with social norms—the age one can marry, or join the military, or retire. Aging is a series of processes that begin with birth and continue throughout the life cycle (Singh and Misra 2009). There is a growing body of evidence that suggests psychological and sociological factors have a significant influence on how individuals age and are significant predictors of functional health and longevity (Singh and Misra 2009).

Aging confronts us with numerous physical, psychological, and social changes that challenge our sense of self and our capacity to live happily. For most seniors retirement years are anticipated positively; responsibilities lessen and opportunities for leisure time increase. Some people experience loneliness and depression as they age as a result of living alone or due to the loss of family members through death, and reduced connections with friends.[1] Rook (1987) found that companionship was a strong buffer for loneliness and stress.

As with all of life's transitions there are discrepancies between what a person expects will happen and what actually happens. Change can bring new challenges and opportunities or frustration and disappointment. With advancing age it is inevitable that people will experience loss, find it difficult to join new social networks, and experience the gradual relinquishment of their autonomy to caregivers on whom they rely for making decisions when they are no longer able to do so (Agich 2003).

[1] See Cacioppo and Patrick (2008) Chap. 6 on understanding how the body experiences the wear and tear of loneliness associated with aging.

J. G. Bruhn, H. M. Rebach, *The Sociology of Caregiving*,
Clinical Sociology: Research and Practice, DOI 10.1007/978-94-017-8857-1_6,

6.2 "Normal" Aging

We are all familiar with comments like, "he (or she) looks younger (or older) than they are (chronologically)." This is because, on the basis of our own experiences in aging and observing the outward signs of aging in others, we have developed stereotypes of what people should look and act like at certain life stages. We then make deductions about how "kind or hard" life has been for them and how well the person has adapted to life changes. Satchel Paige once asked, "How old would you be if you didn't know how old you was?" (Whitbourne 2010). We are all involved in the process of aging. When one is young, aging is associated with growth, maturation and discovery. Some of these facets of aging continue throughout life while others decline. It is tempting to use stereotypes to project our fears and concerns about the challenges of aging. Yet, the effects of aging result from a combination of many factors—genes, lifestyle, and disease all of which can affect the unique ways we age and at what rate. Many of the changes that occur from aging result from gradual losses which begin in early adulthood but their cumulative effects are not recognized until they are seen in the senior years. Therefore, while there are genetic, biological, psychological, and social guidelines or markers which professionals can use to assess our progression in the aging process we cannot reverse the aging process for ourselves or society.

6.2.1 Joann's Longevity

Upon meeting Joann you would likely guess her to be about 65 years old. Widowed for over 20 years, she lives alone in a street level, one bedroom apartment in a large apartment complex and gets around with the assistance of a walker or cane when she remembers. With her selective TV watching of morning game shows and afternoon soap operas, crossword puzzles, table puzzles, playing solitaire on her computer, a voracious appetite for reading, and her frequent phone calls from her daughter and son, she keeps busy, even saving box tops for children in her church's school. Her neighbor picks up her mail from a central mailbox in the complex and her daughter takes her grocery shopping every Tuesday. Her only health problems are minor arthritis in her fingers, recently diagnosed macular degeneration, and sciatica in one leg, so she only has annual medical check-ups and only takes two prescription medications. At 94 years of age her two major worries are whether to sign another 2-year lease for her apartment and her concerns about her son who is in an unhappy marriage and has problems with diabetes and obesity. She is visited twice a month by the pastor and deacon of her church and receives the church newsletter. She goes to bingo events sponsored by her apartment complex, where she plays as many bingo cards as she is permitted. The public library loans her some 11–12 books every month and picks them up and delivers them to her doorstep.

Joann has few visitors, yet is socially connected with her neighbors and can go where she needs to go with the free assistance of Dial-a-ride. She says, "I don't know what I have done to live so long." Yet, she acknowledges that she takes care to eat right, sleep restfully, stays active mentally and physically and maintains her strong spirit. She rarely complains, maintaining an optimistic attitude, and knows her limitations. Recently her daughter and she visited several assisted living facilities to get a feel for cost and suitability. But as Joann says with a smile, "I'm not quite ready for that."

Joann could be considered as an example of "normal" aging. She is an inspiration to those who know her—strong-willed, positive, active, and someone who has established a healthy environment for herself. If she had a car she would be visiting her peers and seniors!

6.2.2 Definition and the Realities of the Senior Years

A senior is a person in the final stage of the life course who is still able to make substantial contributions to society. Old age is a social construct rather than a biological stage, therefore the precise onset of old age varies culturally and historically (Maddox 2000).

The "senior years," or "old age," covers a window of time that is often associated with retirement, e.g. age 65, that may occur prior to or after age 65, or not at all depending on a person's physical and mental abilities, financial resources and culture. The aging process and its effects occur in different ways, in different cultures, and at different speeds for each individual. Caregiving needs change as we age. Usually seniors and their families are not adequately prepared for the changes that accompany increasing age, especially the stresses that accompany caregiving and care receiving. The goal for caregiving in the senior years is to maximize the positive and develop strategies for coping with both stress and loss.

Adult children are the main resources in helping their parents navigate through the senior years. In the absence of a family member to be a caregiver, the senior may have to be cared for in a facility staffed by professional caregivers which will require additional adjustments for the senior. Medicare and Medicaid generally don't provide coverage for informal or custodial caregiving. Therefore, an older spouse, or adult child, or other family member provides the care, covers the cost, and supplies housing for older family members at the level of assistance they need at a given point in the aging process (Brandt 2000).

6.3 Empowerment as a Process

The primary objective of a caregiver is to convey to the care recipient that they have input into decisions that affect their life. Any change is best done with the senior expressing their feelings and preferences, especially when moving from their home to a facility. The lack of opportunity for input can result in the feeling of being placed or put. This can generate a feeling of being abandoned and lead to depression (Brandt 2000). For seniors to relinquish the expression of choice and decision-making is an affront to their independence, identity, and to their self-esteem. Moving is always stressful. The loss of one's home, neighbors, and community can make the senior feel very vulnerable. Studies have shown, for example, that the first year of residence in a nursing home carries the highest risk of death for the resident. While higher rates of death would be expected among the less healthy and frail, there is something about the transfer to a facility and its social ambience that play a role in determining the risk of death for some residents (Reid 2008). Pneumonia is the leading cause of death in facilities where there is also a high risk of contracting an infectious disease.

There are many reasons why a senior may need to be in a structured environment with constant care and surveillance. With progressive aging a point may be reached where health and safety indicate that independent living is no longer possible. There is usually a gradual increase in signs that an alternate arrangement is needed, e.g. falls, car accidents, and neglect in activities of daily living and self-care. It is important that seniors stay physically and mentally active because this has been shown to improve health and longevity. Staying socially connected is important to ward off isolation and depression. If the senior lives alone, caregivers should arrange for transportation for shopping and volunteering. Getting out is important and gives seniors something to look forward to. The challenge for caregivers is to anticipate and recognize the limits of empowerment. Seniors are aware of most changes in their mind and body but may be reluctant to initiate a conversation about it with their caregivers.[2] It often takes the occurrence of negative events such as a fall or car accident before this conversation takes place. It is important that conversations about losses such as leaving one's home or giving up driving a car be done in a way that empowers persons to make some decisions about daily living and maintain their autonomy as long as possible.

Manji and Dunn (2010) observed the living experiences, and interviewed family members and caregivers, of 16 individuals who had developmental disabilities and dementia and lived in a group home. Persons with developmental disabilities were included as they will be predisposed to dementia as the prevalence of dementia is about four times higher among people with developmental disabilities than in the general population. The study identified two social processes: marginalization and supported empowerment.[3] The process of marginalization involves how dementia

[2] One of the biggest misconceptions about dementia is that it is part of the normal course of aging. In a recent survey by the Alzheimer's Foundation of America the majority of caregivers surveyed said that they were aware that Alzheimer's disease has both cognitive and behavioral symptoms but two-thirds (64 %) didn't recognize the behavioral symptoms as problems, believing that they were just a normal part of aging. See "Alzheimer's Caregivers: Behavioral vs. Cognitive Challenges," September 2012. Alzheimer's Foundation of America. Also see, Kiyak et al. (1994). Functional health was consistently rated as more impaired by family caregivers of demented patients than by the patients themselves. The capacity for self-observation is partially preserved in Alzheimer's patients in mild to moderate stages.

[3] Mead (2010). A description of a facility that offers dementia patients a comfortable decline instead of imposing a medical model of care, which seeks to defer death through escalating interventions.

affects people as they incur multiple losses in ability, home, and community. The authors found that, despite these losses, individuals could maintain meaningful connections and participation in a community where supportive empowerment is practiced by the staff and family.

6.4 Successful Aging

The concept of successful aging was introduced by Rowe and Kahn (1998) in the context of separating the effects of disease from the aging process. They proposed that individuals who aged successfully would show little or no age-related decreases in physiological function, while those aging usually would show disease-associated decrements often interpreted as the effects of age. While the idea of successful aging is intriguing, it has been difficult to operationalize. It has been difficult to define successful aging (Strawbridge et al. 1996). Only a small percentage of adults meet Rowe and Kahn's definition suggesting that it is too rigorous for use in public health as a benchmark for measuring and monitoring the health status of the older population (Baltes and Baltes 1990; McLaughlin et al. 2010).

Numerous studies have been conducted to identity the critical elements and a standard definition of "successful aging" (Kahn and Rowe 1987; Vaillant and Mukamal 2001; Depp and Jeste 2009). These studies have often been unidimensional and focused around the physical and cognitive aspects of aging. There is an unstated impression that "successful aging" means the absence of the physical and cognitive diseases of aging. Even when older adults are asked for their views on what constitutes successful aging they favor a multidimensional viewpoint which portrays aging as a process rather than a state to be reached.[4] Young et al. (2009) moves beyond a limited perspective and proposes that successful aging may coexist with diseases and functional limitations if compensatory psychological and social mechanisms are used to adapt to aging. Young and his colleagues suggest three principles of successful aging: the heterogeneity of aging, multiple pathways to successful aging, and individual compensation mechanisms to adjust to aging-related changes. They define successful aging as "*a state wherein an individual is able to invoke adaptive psychological and social mechanisms to compensate for physiological limitations to achieve a sense of well-being, a high self-assessed quality of life, and a sense of personal fulfillment even in the context of illness and disability*" (p. 89).

Young's definition of successful aging is used here as one of the broader definitions in the published literature with one caveat, successful aging is not a fixed state, or level, or point in time that a senior strives to achieve, rather successful aging is a process that changes induced by environmental or personal factors outside of one's

[4] Older adults' definition of successful aging is multidimensional, encompassing physical, functional, psychological and social health. In contrast, none of the published work describing attitudes of successful aging includes all four dimensions. Future work would benefit from an expanded definition to adequately reflect the perceptions of older adults. See Phelan et al. (2004).

control. Kahn and Rowe (1987) refer to such changes as "reductions" in autonomy and control. Possible reductions include physical impairments, reduced economic capability and residential moves which can alter the extent of a senior's autonomy and control. Rowe and Kahn (1998) suggested that factors such as social support and feelings of control might actually slow the biological aging process.

6.4.1 Autonomy and Control

Joann, at age 94, had retained her autonomy and control over her life and lifestyle for the time being. She was anticipating when she might have to permit her daughter to assume responsibility for her finances and provide assistance in her activities of daily living. Research has found that the relinquishment of autonomy and control have adverse effects on individuals' emotional states, performance, well-being, and physical state. Autonomy confers self-esteem and independence. Control provides predictability. Joann talked openly about small changes in her body such as the gradual worsening of her arthritis, the increasing difficulty with her vision, and her hypervigilance about falling, almost wishing that she did not have to live too much longer to experience the cumulative effects of changes that would require that she become dependent on care from others.

6.4.2 Social Support and Social Networks

Autonomy and control are closely tied to the perception and availability of social support and utilization of social networks. Joann has a small but strong, and active social support network. She is in weekly telephone contact with her son and daughter and grandchildren. Neighbors collect her daily mail so she spends the majority of time every day at home entertaining herself. She wears a Life Alert button in case she experiences an emergency.

Research has shown that older people have different social networks to help them feel connected and maintain their sense of well-being (Uchino 2004). Interestingly the volume of contact with people fluctuates with age rather than declining steadily. The oldest-old (ages 75–85), for example, tend to have smaller social networks, have less emotional closeness to network members, and are more likely to socialize with their neighbors, attend church, and volunteer.

Fiori and her colleagues (2006) believe that different networks have different effects on health.[5] The different roles each person plays introduces them to different networks that help them feel socially connected and maintain their sense of well-being. High quality social connections are thought to be associated with better mental

[5] For recent research on the relationships between social support, networks, and happiness see Population Reference Bureau (2009). This newsletter explores the ways social networks affect health and happiness, and influence longevity.

health, while individuals who have fewer more restricted networks are more likely to experience depression. Older individuals from different cultures have different expectations of social support. For example, some cultures expect children to provide social and emotional support for their elderly parents more than other cultures.

As the population ages, more people are reaching old age having lived with a long-term impairment, such as multiple sclerosis or rheumatoid arthritis. Social support is critical in ameliorating the aging experience with a long-term impairment. Casey and Stone (2009) explain that coping with long-term physical impairments may be a lonely experience when the person lacks a strong network of family and friends to offer emotional support as they deal with the long-term changes that occur with these illnesses. Patients with these long-term illnesses stated that their impairments were less stressful when they could share their thoughts, feelings, and problems with others.

6.5 Insights into Long, Happy Lives: The Results of the Harvard Grant Men Study

One of the methodological limitations of studies of aging and longevity is the lack of longitudinal data on individuals as they progress through the life course. The results of a 75 year study of aging, which began in 1938, were recently released (Vaillant 2012). A group of behavioral scientists at Harvard University were interested in identifying predictors of optimal and successful aging in men. W. T. Grant (Grant Foundation) who financed the study, was interested in what makes a good manager or leader. The variables studied were diverse and included childhood environment, genetics, maturation, work, alcohol use and abuse, coping styles, marriage, social support, and participants' greatest joys and regrets.

There were two socially different cohorts: 237 physically and mentally healthy Harvard sophomores from the classes of 1939 to 1944 and a second cohort of 332 disadvantaged non-delinquent inner-city youths who grew up in Boston neighborhoods between 1940 and 1945.

The subjects were all male, white, and of American nationality. The men were followed for 68 years until they reached the age of 70 years for the inner-city group and 80 years for the Harvard cohort. The men were evaluated every 2 years by questionnaires, information from their physicians, personal interviews and interviews with three generations of relatives. The study was described as it progressed in two books by psychiatrist George E. Vaillant (1977, 2002).

The study is still ongoing, but to date there are several findings about healthy and unhealthy male adaptation to life.

- The most important contributor to joy and success in adult life is love, and the second greatest contributor is the individual's involuntary coping styles or defense mechanisms.
- What goes right in childhood predicts the future far better than what goes wrong. A warm childhood predicts joy and success in adult life.

- The capacity for intimate relationships predicts flourishing in all aspects of men's lives.
- Marriages become happier after age 70.
- Alcoholism was the most important cause, not the result, of unhappy marriages.
- As men approach old age, their boyhood relationships with their mothers were associated with their effectiveness at work, continuing to work until age 70, and late-life income. Men's warm relationships with their fathers (but not with mothers) seem to enhance their capacity to play. Good father-son relationships predicted subjective life satisfaction at age 75.
- After age 40, IQ does not count for much.
- Men's military rank once discharged from WWII was significantly correlated with a cohesive home atmosphere in childhood and warm relationships with mother and siblings. Body build, parental social class, endurance on a treadmill, and IQ were not associated with attained military rank.
- Of the 26 personality traits assessed when the men were in college, the one called Practical, Organized best predicted objective mental health at ages 30 through 50.
- Men who live to be 100 years old are usually pretty active at age 95.

Vaillant reviewed the limitations of the 75 year study including its focus on white, educated men and the intellectual interests of the several financial benefactors who underwrote the costs of such a long-term study. Indeed, the study's objectives were tweaked whenever there was a change in the study's leadership, which was about three times over 75 years. Vaillant notes that in retrospect the study would have benefited from participants who were less homogeneous and more diverse in gender, race and ethnicity, and social class. Every research project is a learning experience in retrospect, especially longitudinal ones. Nonetheless, despite its draw backs, the Harvard Grant Study uncovered three major findings which offer opportunities for replication and in-depth study. They are:

1. A warm childhood is the most important predictive factor in successful aging and a bad childhood is not
2. The most important contributor to joy and success in adult life is love
3. Mature defense (coping) mechanisms do not appear to be essential for sustained good health and successful physical aging

6.6 Summary

The senior years are a time of gains and losses; gains in more discretionary time and losses of family and friends. How the aging process has treated us will determine whether the final stage in life is more positive than negative or vice versa. The senior years are a period of time when we are required to make choices about our dependence/independence, disconnectedness/connectedness, and acceptance/denial of the effects of aging on us. The senior years can be a time of challenges and opportunities or frustration and disappointment. As people are living longer these choices are often complicated by finite resources and the degree which a person can function both physically and mentally. While successful aging is usually tied to the number of years lived, it is also tied to our own expectations and satisfactions in life, or expressed in another way, to what extent do we have unfinished business?

Empowerment is an important aspect of aging. Even when caregiving is minimal seniors value the ability to have input into decisions regarding their care, especially if it involves living in a facility. The first year of residence in a nursing home carries the highest risk of death for the resident. The loss of one's home, neighbors and community can make the senior very vulnerable.

Successful aging may coexist with disease and functional limitations. Autonomy and social support are important aspects of successful aging; it has been suggested that control and support have different effects on individuals, but they are thought to enhance longevity and health.

The longest longitudinal study of health, despite its focus on white, educated men, found that the most important contributor to joy and success in adult life is love, and the second greatest contributor is an individual's coping style. The capacity for intimate relationships predicts flourishing in all aspects of men's lives.

6.7 Questions for Discussion

1. Discuss some of the methodological issues in planning and carrying out a long-term longitudinal study of aging.
2. Is there such a thing as "normal" aging? Discuss.
3. How does "empowerment" relate to aging?
4. Discuss why and how autonomy and control are important in aging.
5. Discuss the evidence for social support and social networks in longevity.

References

Agich, G. J. (2003). *Dependence and autonomy in old age: An ethical framework for long-term care* (2nd ed.). New York: Cambridge University Press.

Baltes, P. B., & Baltes, M. M. (Eds.). (1990). *Successful aging: Perspectives from the behavioral sciences*. New York: Cambridge University Press.

Brandt, A. L. (2000). Transition issues for the elderly and their families. http://www.ec-online.net/knowledge/articles/brandttransitions.html. Accessed 15 May 2013.

Cacioppo, J. T., & Patrick, W. (2008). *Loneliness: Human nature and the need for social connection*. New York: W. W. Norton & Co.

Casey, R., & Stone, S. D. (2009). *Aging with long-term physical impairment: The significance of social support*. Poster presented at conference on Health over the life course. University of Western Ontario, London, Ontario, October 14–16, 2009.

Depp, C. A., & Jeste, D. V. (2009). Definitions and predictors of successful aging: A comprehensive review of larger quantitative studies. *Focus: The Journal of Lifelong Learning in Psychiatry, 8*(1), 137–149.
Fiori, K. L., Antonucci, T. C., & Cortina, K. S. (2006). Social network typologies and mental health among older adults. *The Journals of Gerontology Series B: Psychological Sciences and Social Sciences, 61*(1), P25–32.
Kahn, R. L., & Rowe, J. W. (1987). Human aging: Usual and successful. *Science, 237,* 143–149.
Kiyak, H. A., Teri, L., & Borson, S. (1994). Physical and functional health assessment in normal aging and in Alzheimer's disease: Self–reports vs. family reports. *The Gerontologist, 34*(3): 324–331.
Maddox, G. L. (2000). The behavioral and social dynamics of aging well. In B. D. Smedley & S. L. Syme (Eds.), *Promoting health: Intervention strategies from social and behavioral research.* (pp. 322–336). Washington, DC: National Academy Press.
Manji, S., & Dunn, P. (2010). Supported empowerment for individuals with developmental disabilities and dementia. *Journal on Developmental Disabilities, 16*(1), 44–52.
McLaughlin, S. J., Connell, C. M., Heeringa, S. G., Li, L. W., & Roberts, J. S. (2010). Successful aging in the United States: Prevalence estimates from a national sample of older adults. *Journal of Gerontology: Social Sciences, 658*(2), 216–226.
Mead R. (20 May 2013). The sense of ending: A new direction in dementia care. *The New Yorker,* 92–103.
Phelan, E. A., Anderson, L. A., La Croix, A. Z., & Larson, E. B. (2004). Older adults' views of "successful aging"—how do they compare with researchers' definitions? *Journal of the American Geriatric Society, 52*: 211–216.
Population Reference Bureau. (2009). *Today's research on aging, 17,* 1–7.
Reid, R. C. (2008). Quality of care and mortality among long-term care residents with dementia. *Canadian Studies in Population, 35*(1), 49–71.
Rook, K. S. (1987). Social support versus companionship: Effects on life stress, loneliness, and evaluation by others. *Journal of Personality and Social Psychology, 52*(6), 1132–1147.
Rowe, J. W., & Kahn, R. I. (1998). *Successful aging: The MacArthur foundation study.* New York: Pantheon Books.
Singh, A., & Misra, N. (2009). Loneliness, depression, and sociability in old age. *Industrial Psychiatry Journal, 18*(1), 51–55.
Strawbridge, W. J., Cohen, R. D., Shema, S. J., & Kaplan, G. A. (1996). Successful aging: Predictors and associated activities. *American Journal of Epidemiology, 144*(2), 135–141.
Uchino, B. N. (2004). *Social support and physical health: Understanding the health consequences of relationships.* New Haven: Yale University Press.
Vaillant, G. E. (1977). *Adaptation to life.* Boston: Little, Brown.
Vaillant, G. E. (2002). *Aging well.* Cambridge: Harvard University Press.
Vaillant, G. E. (2012). *Triumphs of experience: The men of the Harvard grant study.* Cambridge: Harvard University Press.
Vaillant, G. E., & Mukamal, K. (2001). Successful aging. *The American Journal of Psychiatry, 158*(6), 839–847.
Young, Y., Frick, K. O., & Phelan, E. A. (2009). Can successful aging and chronic illness coexist in the same individual? A multidimensional concept of successful aging. *Journal of American Medical Directors Association, 10*(2), 87–92.
Whitbourne, S. K. (2010). *The search for fulfillment.* New York: Ballantine Books.

Chapter 7
Socioeconomic Status and Caregiving

7.1 Introduction

Socioeconomic status signifies a person's position within systems of inequality in society. These systems are based on the unequal distribution of resources which is a normal part of society. Most Americans usually do not like the idea of "classes" in our society and the topic of class is one of the few remaining taboo topics among Americans. But inequalities exist as a fact of life.

One obvious inequality is income inequality. Some jobs pay better than others, often because of the training, education, and skills needed. Educational attainment is another way we differ; persons with higher levels of education often qualify for better paying jobs and careers. Finally, some occupations confer a certain amount of prestige or status on the position holder. *These three components, income, educational attainment, and occupational prestige, individually or in some combination, are usually used to identify an individual's socioeconomic status (SES).*

In this chapter we will first review the influence of socioeconomic status on aging and disability, then address socioeconomics as the context of caregiving.

7.2 Socioeconomic Status and Aging

Throughout the life course, individuals' socioeconomic status sets the context of their development. In the stages of childhood, household income, parents' education and occupation are related to the child's life chances, social capital, opportunities, and outcomes including their status attainment as adults. With regard to aging, health is a very important outcome. The relationship between socioeconomic status and health is well known. Pearlin et al. (2005, p. 205) reported that "The evidence amassed from large numbers of studies employing a variety of methods leaves no doubt that differences in people's health and well-being correspond to differences in their status locations within systems of inequality." Pearlin and his colleagues set as their task to conceptualize an explanation for the observed relationship between social and economic position and health disparities. They based

J. G. Bruhn, H. M. Rebach, *The Sociology of Caregiving*,
Clinical Sociology: Research and Practice, DOI 10.1007/978-94-017-8857-1_7,

their conceptualization on the effects of inequality over the life course; health consequences that appear in later life are linked to processes and mechanisms that are evident earlier in the life course and are strongly associated with position in the socioeconomic status hierarchy.

One such mechanism is health-related behaviors such as smoking, obesity, unhealthy diet, lack of exercise, and sedentary life, behaviors that are more likely among people in more disadvantaged classes. A second mechanism is exposure to aversive conditions at work and in residential neighborhoods; those in lower social and economic strata are more likely to be exposed to adverse conditions affecting their health. Third, access to health-related information and access to and use of medical care vary by socioeconomic status. Members of lower strata are slower to acquire and slower to act on health related information. And, fourth, differential exposure to stressors and hardships over the life course; the more advantaged societal members may be shielded from stressors, especially continuous financial strain, while others may be readily exposed to stressors that eventually take a toll on health. Those less educated have more difficult work lives, more pressure, and less security. They are likely to have little economic and social capital. Their neighborhoods may provoke safety concerns, contain barriers to obtaining services, create transportation difficulties and all of these "ambient stressors" add to stress (Pearlin et al. 2005, pp. 207–208).

Ongoing or recurring stressors like economic deprivation and financial strain and the experience of repeated discrimination are examples of stressors that are persistent over time and are associated with more health problems (Pearlin et al. 2005, p. 209). Stress proliferation is an important process contributing to later life health outcomes. Stress proliferation is the idea that stressors do not always come one-at-a-time but can come in bunches. Serious stressors can give rise to additional stressors. Financial strain can mean putting off such things as car or house repairs which create more problems later as the consequences of delaying the repair emerge. Financial strain, a major source of stress, may lead to heightened family conflict, increasing the stress burden on those involved. As people remain in disadvantaged statuses, their risk of stressors continues and accumulates having an eventual cumulative effect on their health later in the life course.

Kahn and Pearlin (2006) specifically studied the effects of financial strain over the life course and its relation to health in later life. They noted that higher SES persons are often able to have generally good health well into older ages compared to those of lower socioeconomic strata who are likely to have functional limitations and illness earlier in their life course. They also noted that it is not a matter of specific risk factors, but a matter of the structure and experience of everyday life associated with differences in social and economic status and the stressors that relate to health problems.

For their study, Kahn and Pearlin were able to obtain data from a sample of 1,167 Medicare recipients age 65 or older from the Washington, D. C. Metropolitan area. In face-to-face interviews, respondents described their financial status at various earlier phases of their life course, their childhood, early adulthood (ages 18–35), middle age (ages 35–50) and later (50+). The objective was to identify times of financial strain over the life course. Their study also examined the question of whether earlier hardship exacerbated the effect of later financial conditions or is later hardship independent of earlier conditions. The primary interest was people's health status in later life. As they remarked, "If earlier hardship continues to influence later health even after accounting for economic circumstances at later ages, this would provide evidence that health disparities may stem from prior stressful experiences…." (Kahn and Pearlin 2006, p. 20).

Results showed that many of the elder respondents (53 %) remembered financial hardships in their childhood. These respondents would have spent at least part of their early years during the Great Depression of the 1930s. The respondents' reports also showed that the extent of financial hardship declines with age; 18.7 % reported financial difficulty in midlife (ages 35–50) and 12.5 % in late midlife (ages 50–65). For these respondents, these periods would have been the eras of economic growth of the 1940s–1960s (Kahn and Pearlin 2006, p. 22–23). Twenty-four percent of respondents reported fair to poor health and 46.2 % reported very good or excellent health.

The main purpose of the research of Kahn and Pearlin was the study of people's health in later life and its relationship to finances over the life course. Interested readers are referred to Table 3 of their report. Their analysis clearly showed that "… the greater the persistence of financial strains across the earlier years of the life course, the greater the damage to multiple dimensions of late life health" (p. 24). A history of continuous, ongoing financial strains are damaging to health and more damaging than episodic periods of strain. Chronic stress has later health consequences.

Another question raised by Kahn and Pearlin was whether the stage of life, such as childhood or midlife, in which financial stress occurs leads to different outcomes. Again the analysis clearly showed that the later the life course stage in which financial strain took place, the more effect it had on these elders' health. Analysis also showed that the persistence of strain, the frequency and duration, had significant association with later life health. Early life hardship followed by mid-life and later times of hardship was associated with illness, functional impairment and depression. Continuous or frequently repeated strain appeared to have a cumulative effect on health across the life course.

Luo et al. (2012) studied a different stressor, discrimination, in their research on socioeconomic status and health in later life. As a source of stress, discrimination can take on the characteristics of frequency and persistence of stressors associated with health deficits. And it may be the case that lower status individuals may find themselves more often the targets of discrimination.

For this research, Luo and coworkers took data from the 2006 and 2008 waves of the *Health and Retirement Study* (HRS), a nationally representative sample of older adults that started in the early 1990s and re-interviewed participants every 2 years. There were 6,377 respondents included for this research. Discrimination was measured as both everyday discrimination—disrespect, lack of courtesy, poor services, being treated as dumb—and major discrimination—not hired, not promoted, not qualified for a loan, prevented from moving to a neighborhood.

Results showed that 30% of respondents reported age discrimination, 14% reported gender discrimination and 14% reported racial discrimination. Persons divorced or separated or widowed reported higher levels of everyday discrimination compared to those married or partnered. Older persons were less likely to report discrimination and as age increased, levels of both types of discrimination decreased. Household assets, a measure of socioeconomic status, was inversely related to discrimination; the fewer assets, the more discrimination and the more assets the less reported every day and major discrimination events.

Luo et al. included measures of other stressors including acute and chronic stressors, especially financial strain. Stressors were positively associated with perceived discrimination, both everyday and major discrimination events. That is, people who reported greater stress also reported more discrimination experiences. This could be an example of stress proliferation.

Four health outcomes were part of the analysis: self rated health, functional limitations, chronic conditions, and depressive symptoms. These were assessed for changes over the 2 year period. Older women showed more functional limitations and fewer chronic conditions than men in 2008. Increasing age was generally associated with decline in all three physical health areas. Lower education levels were associated with health decline. Lower household income and lower household assets were both associated with indicators of health decline and everyday discrimination was associated with poorer health for all four indicators at the second interview in 2008. Authors also reported that the number of lifetime discrimination events was associated with more depressive symptoms and marginally significant association with functional limitations. Finally, measures of general stress, which discrimination experience added to, were also related to health decline. Social status and persistent stress affected health.

More useful evidence on aging and health and socioeconomic status comes from earlier research by House et al. (1994) who noted that some segments of the population significantly delay the onset of morbidity and functional limitations and that socioeconomic status is particularly relevant to this. Data was obtained from *The Americans Changing Lives Survey*, a longitudinal study with a national sample of non-institutionalized persons age 25 and older. The initial interviews were conducted in 1986 with a second interview about 2 1/2 years later in 1989. Analysis was based on 2,867 respondents. The outcome studied was respondents' health in terms of chronic conditions and functional ability. Data were also obtained on education and household income as measures of socioeconomic status and on psychosocial characteristics that may be associated with health risks. These included health risk behaviors like smoking, weight, and alcohol use. Psychosocial indicators also included social relationships and supports, acute and chronic stress indicators, and measures of self-esteem and feelings of mastery.

Results showed that gender, age, education, and income were all highly significant predictor's of chronic conditions and functional status. Age was also found to interact with both education and income. Advancing age associated with low income and/or lower education was significantly associated with chronic conditions and functional limitations. The data also provided evidence that persons in the higher income and education segments of society were able to significantly postpone declines in health into middle or early old age. The results supported the authors' view that socioeconomic status is a significant predictor of health changes over the life course and that the mechanism is differential exposure to risk factors and the impact of this exposure on those exposed to those risks. That is, exposure and impact vary by socioeconomic status. And as House et al. (p. 228) pointed out, "The health impact of many risk factors increases in later middle age and early old age thus maintaining their contribution to the social stratification of aging and health."

The researchers reported in the pages above show the connection of socioeconomic status to health generally. Al Hazzouri et al. (2011) specifically focused on dementia, an illness often involving family caregivers. They studied the relationship between life course changes in socioeconomic status, cognitive decline and dementia. They noted that economic position early in the life course may have effects on the brain and cognitive development which may emerge as dementia risk in later life. Data for this research came from the *Sacramento Area Latino Study on Aging* (SALSA), a longitudinal cohort study of Mexican Americans in the Sacramento area who were ages 60–101 at the time of baseline in 1999. Clinical data were collected about once a year over about seven years. Socioeconomic position at three life course stages was determined from interviews. The SES trajectories across life course stages were found to be associated with incidence of dementia/cognitive impairment, not dementia (CIND). That is, the risk of dementia or cognitive impairments was related to the life course of socioeconomic status. Lower status was associated with greater risk of dementia which increased as the extent of time spent in low status increased.

Basu (2013) also directed her research attention specifically to dementia. Her main interest was the relationship between education and dementia, but, as she pointed out, socioeconomic resources during adulthood often account for education. Data for Basu's research came from a sample of persons age 70 or older from the 2000 and 2002 waves of the *Health and Retirement Study* (HRS). These persons were selected based on cognitive scores. Respondents received clinical and neurological evaluations and had a diagnosis of dementia, or Alzheimer's disease, or cognitive impairment not demented (CIND). Baseline data came from the HRS of 1996 and 1998. Measures included the diagnoses, measures of SES, educational attainment, measures of health behaviors, chronic conditions and relevant genetic characteristics. Data also included a family history of memory disorders.

Results showed a strong and significant relationship between education and dementia. In particular, the odds of dementia (vs. CIND or normal cognition) were 14 % less for each additional year of education among these older adults. The odds of developing dementia were 2.29 times higher for Medicaid recipients, eligibility for Medicaid being a marker for low SES. The author concluded, "The association between education and dementia was independent of a wide range of lifestyle and vascular related risk factors…." (Basu 2013, p. 23).

Health in later life, including chronic conditions, functional limitations, and cognitive impairment is strongly related to the need for caregiving. The brief review in the pages above reflects an extensive research tradition that has shown the association between socioeconomic position across the life course and health in later life.

7.3 The Socioeconomic Context of Caregiving

Rapid demographic change has been taking place in the United States affecting the societal context of caregiving. The population, age 65 and older has shown rapid growth; it was 40.3 million in 2010, an increase of over 5 million or 15.1 % since 2000. Persons in the age group 45–64 increased by 33 % and these are people who will reach age 65 sometime in the next two decades (Administration on Aging 2012). People are living longer and therefore more likely to need help with some of the emerging problems and illnesses associated with aging. Other trends, the increasing divorce rate, lower fertility rates, fewer children and smaller families, and the increasing labor force participation of women all potentially reduce the capacity of the informal, family based caregiving system to meet a growing need (Williams et al. 2003, p. 281).

For families that can afford to pay, the market offers an array of services to fill the need for custodial and other home care for family members. For families that cannot afford to pay, family caregivers provide the care services. Use of purchased services is related to ability to pay. Supports from public sources, at this writing, remain unpredictable for most families. As Levine et al. (2006, p. 305) observed, "The United States lacks a comprehensive and coherent long-term public policy for people who are chronically ill, frail, or disabled." In fact, the policy appears to be, "let the family do it." And, "the family" usually means the women, daughters, daughters-in-law, wives, etc.

Saraceno (2010, p. 32) suggested three perspectives on social status; how it affects a person's risk for dependency in later life, how it affects the availability of resources needed to deal with one's dependency, and the impact on the person and those who are the caregivers. The third point is relative to caregivers' resources. In particular, the question was raised about intergenerational transfer of money and person's responsibilities to their aging parents and to their own children. For example, midlife adults may be faced with the unpleasant task of having to decide about devoting savings to their children's education or to the care of elderly parents.

Saraceno's macro-social analysis of modern industrial societies touched on a critical caregiving issue: who pays? Three patterns were identified. The first was labeled *familism by default* (p. 33), a situation in which there are no public programs or funds provided to families or caregivers. The second was labeled, *supported familism*, a situation where families receive assistance in maintaining their financial and their caregiving responsibilities. The third pattern was labeled *defamilization*, the situation where third-party payers—market mechanisms, such as privately purchased services paid for out-of-pocket or by insurance or government programs, take over. Obviously, purchased services will be largely affected by family resources.

As Saraceno noted, the greater the emphasis on *familism by default* the greater the impact of the social and economic status of the family. Saraceno's analysis was confined to the European Union and did not include the United States. But Robinson's analysis (1997, p. 245) would seem to put the U.S. pattern into the *familism by default* category. Her view that, "policy makers place increasing pressure on families to provide care" is certainly consistent with family as the default option. She pointed out that Medicare does not cover home care or custodial needs of the elderly or the chronically ill. The pressure she referred to developed out of emerging concerns for cost containment measures and the politics of federal expenditures for healthcare. Levine et al. (2006, p. 305) pointed out that governments at all levels are moving away from supporting expensive institutional care and toward community-based care with families carrying the load. If Medicare is not a resource, and qualifying for Medicaid requires meeting very stringent conditions, family caregiving becomes the default option and family resources will affect caregiving. Robinson (1997) made the point that family caregiving provides a public benefit. The most obvious benefit is the value of the free labor. It reduces the number of nursing home or other institutional admissions which are often paid for with public funds. And, when elders remain in the community, they purchase goods and services locally. They become impoverished if/when they transfer to institutional care.

Harrow et al. (2004) raised questions about the actual dollar cost for family caregivers of persons with Alzheimer's disease or other dementias. They noted that about two thirds of caregivers use some formal services. They found that higher socioeconomic status was associated with greater likelihood of formal services costs. Care recipient's increasing age was also associated with increasing likelihood of formal services use. And lower mental status scores, poorer care receiver health, and the extent of bothersome care receiver behaviors also increased the likelihood of formal services costs. Formal services costs were also significantly higher for employed caregivers compared to non-employed caregivers.

Many of the formal services used, depending on the state of residence, are not covered by insurance or public programs like Medicaid or Medicare. There is significant state-to-state variation on what is covered. Many services require out-of-pocket expenditures; family caregivers shoulder most of the burden. Harrow et al. estimated the costs to family caregivers for formal services for persons with dementia. They based their estimates on six sites around the country: Birmingham, Boston, Memphis, Miami, Palo Alto, and Philadelphia. The average cost estimate was \$ 672 per month with a high of \$ 1,198 per month in Boston to a low of \$ 497 per month in Memphis. These cost estimates were for services that support family caregiving: homemaker services, delivered meals, transportation services, a visiting nurse, and day care. They do not include physician or other medical care or institutional care. Even at the lowest level these costs could represent a significant financial burden to most family caregivers.

Harrow and colleagues also estimated the dollar value of informal care provided by family caregivers. They obtained data on hours of care provided and on various tasks performed and estimated the dollar value using wage rates appropriate to location and activity. The dollar value (in 1997 dollars) of the free labor of informal caregiving ranged from \$ 2,164 per month in Memphis to \$ 1,816 per month in Philadelphia.

Knickman et al. (2003) applied a simulation model to develop estimates of the ability of elderly persons to pay for healthcare services. Their model, originally developed and refined since 1986, used census data and economic models, "to capture the interaction of demographic and economic factors that affect the resources of the elderly and their use of acute and long-term care services" (p. 169). The model provided projections of costs and projections of ability to pay to 2015 and to 2030. On average the projections of the ability of the elderly and caregivers to provide in-home services are positive. Fewer elders are projected to be in the lowest income category. Real income among the elderly was projected to increase to 2015 and 2030. Liquid assets other than real estate are projected to increase with growth somewhat more rapid to 2015, and slower 2015–2030 (Knickman et al. 2003, pp. 168–170).

One concern expressed by Knickman and his co-authors was the development of multi-tiered healthcare with the wealthy at the top and the poor and middle income people in the lowest tier. They stratified the elderly into three categories based on their ability to handle the costs of catastrophic health events like chronic diseases and long-term care frequently not covered by insurance. The lowest group members, labeled the *Medicaid Bound,* are lower income people who qualify for Medicaid and will need to depend on public sources if available. The highest group labeled the financially independent, are those with adequate resources to pay for discretionary health and preventive services and should be able to afford long-term needs with their current income and/or savings. Those in the middle and working class who do not qualify for Medicaid would have to "spend down," that is, use up savings and assets, to qualify for Medicaid.

Projections showed that the percent of the financially independent tier should grow, the percent of the Medicaid bound decrease and the in-between group stay about the same to 2030. But, while the percentage of the Medicaid bound is projected to decrease, the increase in the number of elders means an increase in the number of those eligible for Medicaid. As the authors pointed out, unless major changes occur in the way healthcare is funded in the United States, stratified healthcare is likely to accelerate. They also expressed concern that the middle and working class elders are at the greatest risk of getting left behind in a multi-tiered system. So, while on average the situation seems positive there is reason for concern for a significant proportion that may have financial problems. Recent data shows that 9.5 % of persons age 55 and over fall below the poverty threshold. The poverty rates are 8.1 % for persons aged 65–74, 9.2 % for persons 75–84, and 12.3 % for persons aged 85 and older (U.S. Census Bureau 2011).

The socioeconomic status of the caregiver and the family is a key factor in the caregiving context. From the perspective of potential care receivers, socioeconomic status across the life course is causally connected to an individual's health and the need for care. From the perspective of the caregiver socioeconomic status is related to the resources they can bring to caregiving including the caregiver's strength, health, resilience, knowledge, skills, and material resources. As Schulz and Sherwood (2008, p. 109) noted low socioeconomic status persons may be more likely to take on the role of caregiver, but their low SES is itself a risk factor for poor health in addition to stressors from caregiving itself.

The transition to the caregiving role involves contextual factors that include socioeconomic status and income as well as education, employment, and other roles, such as parenting, that might coincide with caregiving. Marks et al. (2008) investigated aspects of the transition to filial caregiving. Their data came from the National Survey of Families and Households, a longitudinal study with a nationally representative sample of non-institutionalized adults age 19 and older. Initial interviews were in 1987 and 1988 (time 1) with a second interview approximately 5 years later, 1992–1994 (time 2). The samples for analysis in this study were 1,060 respondents age 25–65 with one parent alive over the course of the study. Outcome measures included mental health, hostility, positive affect, psychological well-being, self-esteem, and self rated health as well as caregiver status at time 2. The researchers were primarily interested in those respondents who began caregiving sometime during the 5 years between interviews.

The research team found that those sons and daughters who became caregivers during this study showed an increase in depressive symptoms compared to those who did not start caregiving. The stress of caregiving was exacerbated by the stress of low income needed to meet increased demand. Low income daughters who began caregiving reported greater physical health declines compared to daughters with higher incomes. But low income daughters had fewer depressive symptoms, less hostility, and better psychological well-being than higher income daughters. Lower income sons who started caregiving also reported higher levels of personal mastery compared to higher income sons. Marks et al. also reported gender differences in response to becoming caregivers. Being employed and caregiving increased hostility and depressive symptoms and decreased psychological well-being more for women than for men. Low income affected women's sense of mastery more than men's.

Considering socioeconomic status, Marks et al. reported that indicators of disadvantaged status—lower income and lower educational attainment—were associated with better well-being for those adult children who entered caregiving. The authors interpreted this as possibly a greater sense of familism—a traditional sense of obligation and responsibility to family and family members—among lower compared to higher socioeconomic status persons.

Kneipp et al. (2004) gave some recognition to family caregiving as a default option and significant public health resource. They also noted that responsibility for informal and custodial care "has increasingly been thrust…onto women" (Kneipp et al. 2004, p. 25). Their point is borne out by data from the National Alliance for Caregiving (NAC 2009, p. 14) which showed that 66 % of caregivers are women. Kneipp et al. also conducted research on the transition to caregiving. Their specific focus was the burden of caregiving experienced by low income women who were making a transition from welfare to work and the combination of caregiving and employment. Caregiver burden is usually defined as the stresses of meeting the demand of caregiving and feelings that arise in response to tasks, physical demands and time taken in caregiving.

Adult child care networks sometimes change over time. Sinovacz and Davey (2007) analyzed changes in adult networks. They noted that changes in family structure may reduce the ability of care networks to provide adequate care. They also noted that those parents with higher socioeconomic status could have greater access to paid services which may reduce the stress of caregiving on their adult children. This, in turn, could mean longer maintenance of care. The study obtained data from 1992–2000 as part of the longitudinal *Health and Retirement Study*. The hypothesis was that there would be less change for parents with higher socioeconomic status based on their ability to obtain formal care. This hypothesis was not supported however. But, if adult children provided financial assistance, caregiver changes were more likely. Generally, the finding was that changes in primary caregiver were less likely for parents with better education but there was no other effect of parents' SES. Authors interpret this as the potentially greater access to paid sources of support may actually facilitate long-term family caregiver support.

As data for their study, Kneipp et al. had a random sample of women in a Florida county drawn from an agency database. Women were age 18 or older, were welfare recipients who had left welfare for a job within the previous year. It is important to note, as the authors did, the jobs that these women leaving welfare found were low-wage with limited flexibility for hours of work, no benefits or paid sick leave or family leave and little opportunity for advancement.

The majority of the respondents (85 %) were employed, working 40 h or more per week and most had at least one child at home. Sixty-three percent of these women were regular caregivers for other family members mostly parents or grandmothers. Thirty percent of respondents reported having to leave a job to provide care. Measures of caregiver burden indicated that the women experienced moderate burden. Though not quite statistically significant, measures of job flexibility and burden showed some association.

Barnes et al. (1995) studied the effects of employment on caregivers. They compared women, daughters who were primary caregivers of their parents. The caregivers were either employed, were never employed, or ended their employment to care for their parent. The criteria for inclusion in the longitudinal study were that the care recipient was age 64 or older and needed help with two or more ADLs/IADLs, and the daughter was the primary caregiver.

The study found that daughters who left employment were more involved with assisting with ADLs than employed daughters. More than the employed and never employed, daughters who quit work helped their parent with self-care, incontinence, mobility, instrumental activities, and healthcare. The researchers assessed caregivers' reaction to caregiving which included measures of caregivers' self-esteem, evaluation of family support, and the impact of caregiving on their health, finances, and schedule. In general no significant differences were found among the groups on these indicators. Also, there were no significant differences in the use of formal services. Caregiving strain was greatest for the women who had quit their jobs. The jobs had provided an income and benefits as well as personal feelings of accomplishment and a source of social interaction with co-workers. For the employed caregivers, the job also offered a respite from caregiving.

What are conditions like for employed caregivers? Lahaie et al. (2012) set out to explore and assess the experiences of employed caregivers. They posed some critical questions for research:

Are working caregivers different from working adults who are not caregivers?
Are there social disparities in the working conditions faced by adult caregivers?
Are there social disparities in the job outcomes of working caregivers?
Are there social disparities in how much caregiving responsibilities affect caregivers' quality of life?

Data for the study reported by Lahaie et al. came from the *Work, Family, and Community Nexus Survey*, a nationally representative sample of U.S. adults, 18–69. The researchers had 2,674 respondents in their analysis sample who were employed full or part-time. The survey assessed working conditions, supportiveness of the workplace, acceptance of workers' small schedule adjustments, formal policies like paid maternal and paternal leave, paid leave to care for family health needs, paid sick days, paid vacation days, unpaid leave to care for family health needs, unpaid personal days, access to medical and hospital insurance, and employee flexibility to set their own schedule and move back and forth from between full-time and part-time. Job outcomes were assessed as wages and wage loss, or job loss, having to quit, being under employed, and changing from full-time. Other measures were quality of life, well-being, and demography.

Results showed that compared to employed non-caregivers a significantly higher percentage of employed caregivers had only a high school education while non-caregivers were significantly more likely to have a college degree. Working caregivers were as likely to be female as male and female caregivers spent an average three more hours per week caregiving. Men were more likely to have the flexibility to change starting times and quitting times as needs arose. Men could also make personal phone calls without consequences. And men were more likely to have paid leave to care for family health needs, paid vacation days, and the ability to take days off without prior permission. Women did have somewhat greater flexibility to switch from full-time to part-time in their same position.

Education made a difference. Employed caregivers with a college degree or more were more likely than caregivers with only a high school education to be able to work from home if necessary. Caregivers with at least a college degree were also more able to make phone calls from work if needed. They were also more able to adjust their work schedule, more likely to have paid leave for family health needs, and paid sick leave.

There were also social disparities in job outcomes for working caregivers. Women caregivers were more likely to report losing income due to caregiving responsibilities, to lose job benefits, and to reduce from full-time to part-time and/or take a less demanding job or quit work entirely in order to meet caregiving responsibilities. However caregivers with at least a college education were significantly less likely to have lost income or have their hours reduced or their job stepped down compared to their counterparts with less education.

Quality of life assessments showed gender differences. Employed women caregivers were more likely to report that caregiving responsibilities interfered with time spent with friends or exercising or participating in education or training opportunities or simply attending to their own emotional needs.

Robison et al. (2009) studied the caregiving experiences of two age cohorts, baby boomers and a preceding, earlier cohort. Their purpose was to study the effects of caregiving such as health, depression, social isolation, and its effects on caregivers' jobs. Data came from a survey of Connecticut residents. One cohort, baby boomers, born between 1946 and 1964 were ages 42–60 at the time of the survey and included 469 caregivers and 1,234 non-caregivers. The older cohort, born prior to 1946, was age 61 and older and included 298 caregivers and 2,040 non-caregivers. Overall 19 % of the total sample were caregiving which was comparable to the national rate. The baby boomers were significantly more likely to be caregivers (61 % vs. 39 %). Caregivers were also significantly more likely to be women and to be employed. About 10 % of both caregivers and non-caregivers reported income inadequacy.

The effects of caregiving studied included depressive symptoms, self rated health, social isolation and dental visits and wellness visits, the latter two as indicators of attention to self-care. Comparison of caregivers and non-caregivers revealed no differences in indicators of depressive symptoms, social isolation, or wellness visits. Caregivers reported better health and were more likely to have dental visits compared to non-caregivers. For caregivers co-residence with care receivers and caring for someone with memory problems predicted depressive symptoms. Caregivers that reported income inadequacy and unmet needs for services had more symptoms of depression. In fact, as reported, caregivers with inadequate income were more than four times more likely to have depressive symptoms.

Caregivers who were employed women often missed work because of caregiving responsibilities and caregivers who reported unmet needs for services missed work about twice as often as others who thought services needs were adequately met. Living with the care recipient predicted social isolation which was felt more strongly if unmet needs for long-term care services were also reported. Employed caregivers reported significantly better health than those not employed though those caregivers who reported income inadequacy were likely to report their health poorer than those with adequate income.

Overall, the study by Robison et al. connected the effects of an important socioeconomic factor like income with services adequacy and adverse effects on caregivers. The obvious strategy to deal with needs for income is employment and many—mostly women—are employed.

Pavalko and Woodbury (2000) had data from two waves, 1987 and 1989, of the *National Longitudinal Survey of Mature Women*, a nationally representative sample of women between ages 30 and 44 when the study survey began in 1967. The sample that Pavalko and Woodbury had for analysis had 2,929 women ages 50–65. The sample included women who started caregiving, women who stopped caregiving, those who were continuing caregiving, and non-caregivers. The study found that women who had been caregivers at the outset of this study (1987) reported significantly more psychological distress and significantly more physical limitations. The highest levels of distress were found among the women with long term caregiving. Baseline measures suggested a connection to caregiving.

Physical limitations were particularly high among the women who stopped caregiving suggesting there may have been a connection. Women who started caregiving during this study period also showed an increase in physical limitations. And, the women who had stopped caregiving continued health declines for a long time after stopping caregiving. Being employed did not affect the likelihood of the women starting caregiving though it was associated with the likelihood of continuing in employment. Of those who ceased employment few also stopped caregiving.

Comparison of caregivers with non-caregivers showed greater increases in physical limitations by caregivers. The pattern observed was increases in physical limitations after starting caregiving but leveling off as the women adapted to continued caregiving. The pattern for psychological distress was that it accumulated; it increased the longer one continued in caregiving.

Pavalko and Woodbury concluded that health may be a factor in women's selecting employment. However, employment may be a buffer. Women who were not employed who started caregiving had greater increases in physical limitations. Women who were continuously employed showed little variation in changes in health suggesting employment as a protective factor. It may be that employed women have additional sources of help including formal services, which employment helps them to afford, and employment may provide a respite from caregiving.

Flaskerud and Lee (2001) noted that the availability of resources plays a significant role in the health of caregivers who are primarily women. They also noted that women's poverty, unemployment, low pay jobs and often lower levels of educational attainment represent a lack of resources including social capital and power that increase women's vulnerability and is linked to poor health. As caregivers this means that women have fewer connections, lack financial resources, and have limited access to community resources to provide additional support for caregiving and to deal with the sources of caregiver burden and stress that are associated with health decline.

Flaskerud and Lee studied two samples of caregivers in southern California conducting in-depth interviews they reported as lasting two to three hours. Respondents were 36 women who were caregivers of persons with HIV/AIDS (PWHA) and 40 women who were caregivers of persons with age related dementia (PWARD). The outcomes studied were a measure of depressive symptoms (CES-D) and self reported health. Some descriptive measures included years of caregiving, hours per day spent caregiving, and functional status and problem behaviors of care recipient, all sources that elevate caregiver burden and have been shown in the past to be associated with declines in caregiver health.

First, Flaskerud and Lee found that the two groups were significantly different with regard to indictors of socioeconomic status. There were significant differences in income and educational attainments among caregivers; caregivers of persons with age related dementia had higher average incomes and higher educational levels. It appeared that the health condition requiring care and the caregiver-care receiver dyad was almost a marker for SES. There were significant differences in caregivers' self-rated health. Caregivers for PWHA rated their health as poorer than caregivers for PWARD. There was also a significant difference in measures of depressive symptoms with caregivers of PWHA significantly higher than caregivers for PWARD. There were also significant differences in emotional responses.

Caregivers of PWHA were angrier, more anxious, more fearful, nervous, and tense, and more irritable. Authors also report the principle conclusion, "…resource variables…contributed the most to the explanation of health status in this sample of caregivers" (Flaskerud and Lee 2001, p. 66).

Wakabayashi and Donato (2005) studied caregiving women's employment from the perspective that caregiving would have adverse effects on women's hours on the job and on their income. They had data from two waves, 1987–1988 and 1992–1994, of the National Survey of Families and Households, a longitudinal study with a representative sample. Their analysis sample included 2,638 women ages 19–70 years old who were in the workforce and working for pay, and had at least one living, not co-resident, parent at the time of both interviews.

Analysis compared various caregiving statuses—those who were not caregivers, those who started, those who continued, and those who stopped caregiving. Women involved in caregiving were a bit older than women who were non-caregivers at both interviews. Women who stopped caregiving had lower educational attainment compared to non-caregivers. Those who continued were less likely to have young children.

When groups were compared by hours at employment, non-caregivers had more hours than women who had started caregiving during the period of the study. Additionally, women who stopped caregiving during the study period earned less than non-caregivers. Those who had been caregivers at the start and continued caregiving over this study earned more by the end of the study period. Age and education interacted with caregiving. Generally older women and women with less education were more likely to experience reduction in hours worked. Results also showed that women who began caregiving had a significantly greater likelihood of leaving the workforce compared to non-caregivers.

In addition to hours worked, Wakabayashi and Donato analyzed respondents' earnings as it related to their caregiving trajectory. They reported that most of the women experienced large reductions in hours worked and in income if they started caregiving during the study period. Again, age and education were factors. Older (age 46+) and younger (19–25) women and those with less than a high school education had large reductions in hours worked if they started caregiving. And lowered hours led to lowered earnings.

Wakabayashi and Donato concluded that women taking on the caregiving role experienced substantial loss of earnings, an issue that needs to be addressed by public policy since family caregiving and the free labor associated with it is the default plan in the absence of any systematic plan for and caring for those who need it. These authors also questioned: What effect does caregiving have on women's retirement income given that pensions and Social Security are determined by earnings; does it contribute to elderly poverty rates? (Wakabayashi and Donato 2005, p. 484)

Wakabayashi and Donato addressed the latter question in a subsequent study (Wakabayashi and Donato 2006). If caregiving reduces women's income, could the effects accumulate over time increasing women's risk of poverty in later life? Data for this study came from the 1991–1992 and 1999–2000 panels of The Health and Retirement Survey. The sample for analysis included 685 women who had at least one living parent in 1992. They were age 65 or older in 2000. The basic outcome showed that those women who receive public assistance or qualify for Medicaid at the second panel in 1999 were highly likely to have been caregivers at the time of the 1991–1992 panel. The authors reported, "Women living in poverty households in 1999 were almost twice as likely as non-poverty women to have been caregivers in 1991…." An interesting additional finding was that the women in poverty or receiving public assistance at the 1999 panel had averaged more hours per week actively caregiving then their counterparts not in poverty. Poor women also worked fewer hours per week and were likely to rate their health as poor compared to non-poor women.

Overall Wakabayashi and Donato concluded that taking on the caregiver role worsened women's economic well-being. Specifically they found that "caregivers who spent 20 h a week assisting their parent with personal care were 25 % more likely than non-caregivers to live in poverty, 27 % more likely to be recipients of public assistance and 46 % more likely to receive Medicaid 8 years later" (Wakabayashi and Donato 2006, p. 268). In addition, their results showed caregiving adversely affected caregivers' health and employment. These costs are borne by caregivers, predominantly women, as a consequence of the U.S. familism by default.

7.4 Summary

A "Perfect Storm" is brewing. The population percentage and the absolute numbers of persons age 65 and older and persons 85 and older have increased significantly in recent decades. At the same time, marriage and childbearing have been delayed, families have become smaller, often geographically dispersed, and women's labor force participation has greatly increased. These social patterns foretell an impending shortage of a caregiving workforce. Yet a pattern of *familism by default* appears to have emerged as the de facto system of care for the chronically ill and for those elders who require care. Employed women have been the primary caregiving workforce providing non-institutional care, sometimes assisted by in-home services providers for those who could afford to purchase these services. However, as Bookman and Kimbrel (2011, p. 117) wrote, many middle and lower income families cannot afford the supportive services that let elders age at home and avoid more costly institutional care.

Projections predict that, on average, the economic situation for elders will improve, possibly making care more affordable for many. But, many of middle income and working class status whose incomes cannot qualify for subsidies like Medicaid, will still be unable to afford services. Workplaces, especially those of the working poor and working class, have not been particularly caregiver friendly. Though there has been some movement in the appropriate direction, especially for larger companies, caregiver friendly jobs have not become the norm.

Those with wealth and assets will be able to control the context of caregiving within their families and respond to needs as they arise. At issue is care for those of middle, working, and lower class status. What appears to be needed is a plan for an organized societal response to the need. Though a largely political debate will probably need to precede a plan, what we do and how we do it—indeed, whether we do it—will show what kind of society we are.

7.5 Questions for Discussion

1. What does the strong relationship between health and socioeconomic status mean for caregiving and why? How does this relationship affect the caregivers?
2. What is "familism by default?" What events, conditions, or other indicators support the view that this is the U.S. pattern of caregiving. What events, conditions, or other indicators provide evidence that this is not the case in the U.S.?
3. What are the social, economic, historical, and cultural factors that have produced the fact that about two-thirds of caregivers are women?
4. How much and to what extent should government programs be instituted to provide for the emerging "perfect storm" mentioned in the conclusion of the chapter. Provide the rationale for your answer.

References

Administration on Aging Administration for Community Living US Department of Health and Human Services Profile of Older Americans: 2012. Administration on Aging, Administration for Community Living, & U.S. Department of Health and Human Services. (2012). *A Profile of Older Americans.*

Al Hazzouri, A. Z., Haan, M. N., Kalbfleisch, J. D., Galea, S., Lisabeth, L. D., & Aiello, A. E. (2011). Life course socioeconomic position and incidence of dementia and cognitive impairment without dementia in older Mexican Americans: Results from the Sacramento area Latino study on aging. *American Journal of Epidemiology, 173*(10), 1148–1158.

Barnes, C. L., Given, B. A., & Given, C. W. (1995). Parent caregivers: A comparison of employed and not employed daughters. *Social Work, 40*(3), 375–381.

Basu, R. (2013). Education and dementia risk: Results from the aging demographics and memory study. *Research on Aging, 35*(1), 7–31.

Bookman, A., & Kimbrel, D. (2011). Families and elder care in the Twenty-First Century. *The Future of Children, 21*(2), 117–138.

Flaskerud, J. H., & Lee, P. (2001). Vulnerability to health problems in female informal caregivers of persons with HIV/AIDS and age-related dementias. *Journal of Advanced Nursing, 33*(1), 60–68.

Harrow, B. S., Mahoney, D. F., Mendelsohn, A. B., Ory, M. G., Coon, D. W., Belle, S. H., & Nichols, L. O. (2004). Variation in the cost of informal caregiving and formal service use for people with Alzheimer's disease. *American Journal of Alzheimer's Disease and Other Dementias, 19*(5), 299–308.

House, J. S., Lepkowski, J. M., Kinney, A. M., Mero, R. P., Kessler, R. C., & Herzog, A. R. (1994). The social stratification of aging and health. *Journal of Health and Social Behavior, 34*(3), 213–234.

Kahn, J., & Pearlin, L. I. (2006). Financial strain over the life course and health among older adults. *Journal of Health and Social Behavior, 47*(1), 17–31.

Kneipp, S. M., Castleman, J. B., & Gailor, N. (2004). Informal caregiving burden: An overlooked aspect of the lives and health of women transitioning from welfare to employment. *Public Health Nursing, 21*(1), 24–31.

Knickman, J. R., Hunt, K. A., Snell, E. K., Alecxlh, L. M., & Kennell, D. L. (2003). Wealth patterns among elderly Americans: Implications for health care affordability. *Health Affairs, 22*(3), 168–174.

Lahaie, C., Earle, A., & Heymann, J. (2012). An uneven burden: Social disparities in adult caregiving responsibilities, working conditions, and caregiver outcomes. *Research on Aging, 35*(3), 243–274.

Levine, C., Albert, S. M., Hokenstad, A., Halper, D. E., Hart, A. Y., & Gould, D. A. (2006). "This case is closed": Family caregivers and the termination of home health care services for stroke patients. *The Milbank Quarterly, 84*(2), 305–331.

Luo, Y., Xu, J., Granberg, E., & Wentworth, W. M. (2012). A longitudinal study of social status, perceived discrimination, and physical and emotional health among older adults. *Research on Aging, 34*(3), 275–301.

Marks, N. F., Lambert, J. D., Jun, H., & Song, J. (2008). Psychosocial moderators of the effects of transitioning into filial caregiving on mental and physical health. *Research on Aging, 30*(8), 358–389.

National Alliance for Caregiving, & AARP. (2009). *Caregiving in the U.S. 2009*. MetLife Foundation.

Pavalko, E. K., & Woodbury, S. (2000). Social roles as process: Caregiving careers and women's health. *Journal of Health and Social Behavior, 41*(2), 91–105.

Pearlin, L. I., Schieman, S., Fazio, E. M., & Meersman, S. C. (2005). Stress, health, and the life course: Some conceptual perspectives. *Journal of Health and Social Behavior, 46*(2), 205–219.

Robinson, K. M. (1997). Family caregiving: Who provides the care, and at what cost? *Nursing Economics, 15*(5), 243–247.

Robison, J. R., Fortinsky, R., Kleppinger, A., Shugrue, N., & Porter, M. (2009). A broader view of family caregiving: Effects of caregiving and caregiver conditions on depressive symptoms, health, work, and social isolation. *Journal of Gerontology: Social Sciences, 64B*(6), 788–798.

Saraceno, C. (2010). Social inequalities in facing old-age dependency: A bi-generational perspective. *Journal of European Social Policy, 20*(1), 32–44.

Schulz, R., & Sherwood, P. R. (2008). Physical and mental health effects of family caregiving. *Journal of Social Work Education, 44*(3), 105–113.

Szinovacz, M. E., & Davey, A. (2007). Changes in adult caregiver networks. *The Gerontologist, 47*(3), 280–294.

U.S. Census Bureau. (November 2011). *Current Population Survey, Annual Social and Economic Supplement*. https://www.census.gov/hhes/www/poverty/publications/pubs_cps.html. Accessed 10 December 2013.

Wakabayashi, C., & Donato, K. M. (2005). The consequences of caregiving: Effects on women's employment and earnings. *Population Research and Policy Review, 24*, 467–488.

Wakabayashi, C., & Donato, K. M. (2006). Does caregiving increase poverty among women in later life? Evidence from the Health and Retirement Survey. *Journal of Health and Social Behavior, 47*(3), 258–274.

Williams, A. M., Forbes, D. A., Mitchell, J., Essar, M., & Corbett, B. (2003). The influence of income on the experience of informal caregiving: Policy implications. *Health Care for Women International, 24*, 280–291.

Chapter 8
Ethnic Variations in Caregiving

8.1 Introduction

Ethnic diversity is a fact of contemporary American society. In this chapter we will explore relationships between ethnic variation and caregiving. First we will look at some relevant population data to outline the scope of the issue. Then we will show how cultural norms shape an important aspect of the context of caregiving. Third, we will offer a perspective for analysis, the stress process model, and then use it to discuss further relationships between ethnicity and caregiving.

8.1.1 Growing Ethnic Diversity

Many ethnic streams have contributed to the diverse population of the United States. The 2010 Census results are summarized in Table 8.1.

As the 2010 Census showed, groups traditionally referred to as ethnic minorities had high growth rates over the decade since the 2000 Census. The earliest immigrant streams were primarily Western Europeans. Another major influx occurred toward the end of the nineteenth Century and early twentieth Century, people came from Eastern and Southern Europe—Italians, Poles, Jews, Russians, Greeks, etc.—and Ireland. From 1860 to the decennial census of 1920, foreign-born constituted about 14 % of the population compared to about 4.7 % in the Census of 1970.

The new immigration, which began to show up in the 1980 Census, represented more people from Latin America and Asia. In 2010, foreign-born represented about 13 % of the population. Table 8.2 shows the new immigration. Immigrants from Europe made up over half of the foreign-born in 1970, compared to about 12 % more recently. This is accompanied by significant immigration from Asia and Latin America. The data show growing diversity within the U.S. and diversity no longer simply means Black and White.

Aging is closely associated with disability and caregiving. In 2000, about 41 million people were age 62 and older, 14.7 % of the population. In 2010, this increased to about 50 million, 16.2 % of the population, a 15 % increase. Compared to younger

J. G. Bruhn, H. M. Rebach, *The Sociology of Caregiving*,
Clinical Sociology: Research and Practice, DOI 10.1007/978-94-017-8857-1_8,

Table 8.1 2010 Census results; percents of population and percent change by race/ethnicity. (Source: U.S. Census Bureau 2012a)

	Non Hispanic white	African American	Native American & Alaska native	Asian American	Native Hawaiian/ Pacific islander	Other	Two or more races	Hispanic/ Latino
2010 Census % of population	72.4	12.6	0.9	4.8	0.2	6.2	2.9	16.3
Percent change 2000–2010	+5.7	+12.3	+18.4	+43.3	+35.4	+24.4	+32.0	+43.0

Table 8.2 Foreign-born population by region of birth, 1970 and 2010. (Source: U.S. Census Bureau 2012)

	1970	1970	1990	1990	2010	2010
	Number × 1,000	Percent	Number × 1,000	Percent	Number × 1,000	percent
Total	9,619	100.0	19,767	100.0	39,956	100.0
Africa	80	0.8	364	1.8	1,607	4.0
Asia	825	8.6	4,979	25.2	11,284	28.2
Europe	5,741	59.7	4,350	22.0	4,817	12.1
Latin America & Caribbean	1,804	18.8	8,407	42.5	21,224	53.1
Mexico	760	7.9	4,298	21.7	11,711	29.3
Other Central American	114	1.2	1,133	5.7	3,053	7.6
South American	255	2.6	1,037	5.2	2,730	6.8
Caribbean	675	7.0	1,938	9.8	3,731	9.3
Other, not reported	1,168	12.1	1,665	8.4	1,024	2.5

groups, older groups showed faster growth rates. Table 8.3 shows age by race/ethnicity. The Table demonstrates that minorities in the U.S. follow the general trend of older persons as a growing segment of the population including the older old, persons aged 85 and older.

The Census Bureau reported that, in 2010, there were 40.4 million persons aged 65 and over, 39.1 million were non-institutionalized. Of the non-institutionalized, 36.7 % or about 14.4 million were listed as "with any disability" (U.S. Census Bureau 2012). Table 8.4 summarizes the extent of difficulty and limitation by race/ethnicity. The Table refers to "complex activity limitations" which means "having one or more of the following limitations: self-care (activities of daily living or instrumental

Table 8.3 Percentage of older adults by race/ethnicity 2000 and 2009. (Source: U.S. Census Bureau 2012)

	Non-Hispanic whites		Black or African American		Hispanic American		Asian American		Total	
Ages	2000	2009	2000	2009	2000	2009	2000	2009	2000	2009
55–59	5.4	7.1	3.7	5.3	2.7	3.6	4.2	5.6	4.8	6.2
60–64	4.4	6.1	3.0	3.9	2.1	2.6	3.3	4.4	3.8	5.2
65–69	3.9	4.6	2.5	2.8	1.7	1.8	2.6	3.1	3.4	3.8
70–74	3.8	3.5	2.1	2.1	1.4	1.4	2.1	2.4	3.1	2.9
75–79	3.2	2.9	1.6	1.6	0.9	1.1	1.5	1.8	2.6	2.4
80 84	2.2	2.4	1.0	1.1	0.5	0.7	0.8	1.2	1.8	1.9
85 & older	1.9	2.4	0.9	0.9	0.4	0.7	0.6	1.1	1.5	1.8

Table 8.4 Percents, basic action difficulty and complex activity limitations by race/ethnicity, 2000 and 2012. (Source: National Center for Health Statistics (NCHS) 2012)

	Anglo American		African American		Asian American		Hispanic American	
	At least one basic action difficulty							
	Age 18–64	Age 65+	Age 18–64	Age 65+	Age 18–64	Age 65+	Age 18–64	Age 65+
2000	21.8	58.0	22.9	60.4	12.6	44.7	16.6	61.5
2010	25.1	59.2	28.6	63.2	12.8	50.1	21.2	61.5
	At least one complex activity limitation							
	Age 18–64	Age 65+	Age 18–64	Age 65+	Age 18–64	Age 65+	Age 18–64	Age 65+
2000	10.1	32.5	11.7	40.3	3.6	nd	7.3	32.4
2010	12.5	31.1	17.3	40.0	5.0	26.7	7.9	37.6

activities of daily living), social or work" (NCHS 2012, p. 201). Basic action difficulties refer to "movement, sensory (seeing or hearing), or cognitive difficulties." Table 8.5 provides some data on rates of disability and need for assistance. Table 8.6 offers some comparisons among groups.

The trends show an increased proportion of the population aging as well as increased ethnic diversity within the United States. And, what is true in general seems to be true as well for ethnic groups within the population. However, minority groups generally show somewhat higher rates of action difficulty, limitations, and disability compared to non-Hispanic whites who show significant advantage in socio-economic status and life chances, including better health and higher life expectancy.

Race/ethnicity and minority group status in the United States is often a marker for the unequal distribution of resources and life chances including life expectancy, health, and access to quality healthcare. As such, race/ethnicity along with educational attainments, household income, and socioeconomic status are life course contextual factors with significant effects on development in general and transition to the caregiving role in particular (Marks et al. 2008).

Ethnicity, as a factor setting the context of caregiving also distinguishes groups on the basis of each group's history and language as well as cultural values, beliefs,

Table 8.5 Degree of disability in U.S. population by race and Hispanic origin, 2010. (Source: U.S. Census Bureau 2012)

		Any disability		Severe disability		Needs assistance	
		Number × 1,000	%	Number × 1,000	%	Number × 1,000	%
Anglo American	Age 15 or older	36,129	22.1	24,669	15.1	8,325	5.1
	Age 65 or older	14,984	48.5	10,789	35.0	4,598	14.9
African American	Age 15 or older	6,967	23.8	5,180	17.7	1,626	5.6
	Age 65 or older	1,897	57.2	1,469	44.3	611	18.4
Hispanic American	Age 15 or older	5,429	15.8	3,795	11.0	1,374	4.0
	Age 65 or older	1,377	52.2	1,124	42.6	493	18.7

Table 8.6 U.S. income, education, and poverty status by race/ethnicity, 2010. (Source: U.S. Census Bureau 2012)

	Total population	Anglo-American	Black/African American	Asian American	Hispanic American
Median family income	63,331	56,178	33,137	66,286	38,818
Percent, families below poverty threshold	16.8	9.9	27.4	12.2	26.5
Percent, high school graduate or higher	85.3	87.6	84.2	85.3	62.9
Percent, college graduate or higher	27.9	30.3	19.8	49.7	13.9

customs, practices, normative expectations, and the intergenerational transmission of these shared elements. The terms *race* and *ethnicity* stand for a set of potential differences in culture, beliefs, practices, opportunities, and resources that affect the context of caregiving. Research on caregiving has recognized this trend and has tried to describe the influence of race/ethnicity on disability and caregiving. Our purpose in this chapter is to review this research. Our generalization is that caregiving is significantly related to the cultural base of the caregivers and care receivers.

8.1.2 A Norm of Family Caregiving & Filial Piety

Pinquart and Sorensen (2005) called attention to cultural norms as they relate to the context of caregiving. They noted that Western cultures emphasize individualism, but ethnic minorities place a higher value on collectivism which includes one placing family ahead of self. The context of caregiving includes norms of duty to care for disabled or elderly, frail or disabled family members. Compared to non-Hispanic whites, racial/ethnic minorities have shown a greater sense of family obligation in caring for elderly and disabled family members. Pinquart and Sorensen (2005) did a meta-analysis of 116 studies of caregiving. Their results showed that minority caregivers had stronger beliefs of filial obligation and a stronger traditional caregiving ideology that emphasized younger generations' duties to family and obligation to care for family members, especially disabled and older members. They also found that, as a result of these cultural beliefs, African American and Latina caregivers received more support from family members compared to Anglo caregivers.

Dilworth-Anderson and Gibson (1999) noted African American cultural values required placing family ahead of individual members and expressing compassion and sensitivity in family interaction. They also noted that ethnic minority families provide most of the care of older members with dementia and that cultural values like inter-dependency of family members, sharing resources, and the centrality of religion shape kin networks of care. Elderly and dependent members become absorbed into these networks. Dilworth-Anderson and Gibson also reported that Hispanics, Native Americans, and Asian Americans, though more diverse than African-Americans, also adhere to these family centered values, that family loyalty and placing the group before the individual member create strong support systems of multiple caregivers for dependent persons and elders.

Bullock et al. (2003) reported that family is an adaptive mechanism for African-Americans whose coping with limited resources has been enhanced by relying on inter-dependence and mutual support in an environment of racism and ethnic stratification. The normative expectation of care given to the old or disabled and the sense of filial obligation and responsibility emerged from the pattern of reliance on family.

Horowitz and Reinhard (1995) compared caregiving networks of white and black families providing care for their adult child with a serious mental illness. Results illustrated the nature of African American care structures. Black parents as caregivers had more extensive ties to extended family members and generally that there was a greater sense of family responsibility and obligation compared to the white families. Black parent-caregivers were able to count on support and assistance from their adult siblings and from extended family members. However, caregiving for the seriously mentally ill adult child was largely confined to the parents among the white families (Horowitz and Reinhard 1995, p. 143).

Puerto Rican care structures differed from those of both blacks and whites. Hinojosa et al. (2009) conducted a longitudinal study in which they compared Puerto Ricans, African-Americans, and non-Hispanic whites who were providing post-acute care for stroke survivors. These authors reported that the collectivist orientation of Hispanic culture resulted in multiple caregivers from a network of nuclear and extended family caregivers. The collectivist orientation included strong loyalty and an obligation to provide support, mostly by women. African American care structures were found to be larger than those of whites and were more likely to include friends and neighbors. Whites had smaller, less diverse care structures, more often a single primary caregiver. Puerto Rican networks were found to be larger than those of blacks and whites and less likely to include non-nuclear family members.

Borrayo et al. (2007) studied Hispanic Americans' beliefs about the caregiver role. They found that home– and family-centered care were a culturally embedded value; that caregiving showed loyalty and solidarity to an older relative. The cultural expectation among Mexican Americans is also that women are expected to be primary caregivers. The value, based on *marianismo,* is the expectation that women are to be nurturing, self-sacrificing, and caring. Authors Borrayo et al. saw this as letting others, especially men, off the hook and placing an unequal burden of familism on Latina caregivers.

Borrayo et al. also noted the lack of a Spanish term directly translatable as "caregiver" in the sense that we have been applying the term here as a specialized—not ordinary—role. The absence of the specific label can be interpreted to mean that caregiving is assumed to be part of regular family roles and that care of elders and disabled family members is an expected part of regular family activities, nothing out of the ordinary.

Weng and Nguyen (2011) studied cultural issues among Asian Americans related to caregiving. This is quite a diverse group that includes Chinese, Japanese, Koreans, Filipinos, Indians, Pakistanis, Vietnamese, etc. What these groups shared was a likelihood of providing care for elderly family members—43 % compared to 19 % of whites—and a sense of obligation to provide caregiving—73 % compared to 43 % of whites. Generally these Asian cultures are family centered and share the collectivist orientation that includes filial piety, a part of which is the value obligation to care for elderly parents and that duty to family is paramount. But, as Weng and Nguyen noted, Americanized children may adopt Western ideas of individualism, individual achievements, and individual happiness and need satisfaction, independence, autonomy from parents, and self support. They may also focus on nuclear rather than extended families. All of this is the opposite of the collectivist ideas that family interests supersede individual interests.

Lai (2010) surveyed Chinese caregivers of elderly family members in Calgary, Canada. He noted that, in the Chinese culture, filial piety, respect for and caring for older family, is an obligation and, traditionally, is a highly regarded belief and practice. It is the collectivist orientation; children are expected to forgo their own interests and place the benefit and well being of parents and family as a priority. It includes financial support and housing elderly parents if necessary. Lai found that the more caregivers identified with filial piety the more they will have a positive outlook on caregiving.

Kimura and Browne (2009) conducted focus groups among Filipino Americans in Hawaii to examine attitudes toward caregiving and services use. Familism and filial piety were central cultural ideas with this group as with other Asian groups. Respondents strongly agreed that care of elders and frail persons was the family's responsibility. Respondents did note that values were changing among the younger, U.S. raised, generation. Though respondents felt that care was the family's responsibility, they were open to community healthcare services and government financial assistance, though less open to formal care services.

Radina et al. (2009) included both extent of family orientation and generation since immigration in their study of how Mexican American caregivers make decisions about providing care and using formal services. Implicit or explicit decision making may be related to orientation to family and extent of acculturation. The cultural preference among Latinos is that care for elders should occur within the family rather than within formal services such as nursing homes. Caregivers play a role in the extent to which older persons use these services either as decision makers or as participants in the decision making process.

The collectivist cultural values may be an important factor in the course and setting of care. Specifically the use of formal and institutional services may be affected. The cultural preference that care should be provided within the family may limit use of outside services (Radina et al. 2009). Herrera et al. (2008) reported that Mexican Americans preferred giving and receiving care in the family context. This was associated with low rates of use of formal, non-family care services including long-term institutional care. Horowitz and Reinhard (1995) noted that African Americans' greater reliance on extended family ties may delay use of formal services until the disorder becomes severe and comes to the attention of agents of social control.

Min and Barrio (2009) compared Mexican Americans and non-Hispanic whites. In their sample, 74.3 % of Latino compared to 32.6 % of Anglo elderly agreed that care should be provided by family members, not outsiders. Also 31.5 % of Latinos in their sample, compared to 73.4 % of Anglos agreed with the idea that it was alright for adult children to place their elderly parents in nursing homes for proper care. These results illustrate cultural beliefs and preferences.

Korean-Americans may benefit from a collectivist orientation in that caregivers may receive support from the family network. However it can hinder the use of professional help. In Korean culture, dementia is regarded as a normal part of aging though it is considered pathology among Anglos. But the Korean American caregivers were not comfortable with outside help. The norm was that a demented parent or spouse was to be kept at home (Lee and Bronstein 2010).

Kimura and Browne (2009) found low use of formal services like adult day care, home health, respite care, and case management by Filipinos in Hawaii. This is consistent with an earlier report (Pinquart and Sorensen 2005) that Asian Americans used fewer formal supports than Anglos. Among Filipinos, the culture requires family care for elderly parents or other older or frail family members. Attitudes toward formal services use was influenced by cultural values and expectations that spouses or adult children should provide care. And there was concern that, for example, a family member would be embarrassed for a stranger to help with bathing.

Lai (2010) also reported that filial piety may have been a key reason why Chinese family caregivers did not use formal and professional services. They were concerned about the cultural expectation; use of formal services could be perceived as evasion of one's responsibility and involved losing face. As Lai reported, both caregivers and care receivers perceived formal services use as losing face (p. 216). The cultural belief was associated with under use of professional services and supports. But formal services were used when the situation got out of hand. Kimura and

Browne (2009) told of one respondent who reported finally placing her husband in a nursing home when her health declined and he needed 24 h care and supervision.

Kimura and Browne said they expected Filipino culture to be a barrier to services use. That was not what they found. Though cultural beliefs may have contributed to low services use there were other significant barriers. Many, especially immigrants, may not have been aware of the services or how to access them. Services were often unavailable or lacked staff to provide them adequately. Discrimination, disrespect and cultural insensitivity often kept people away. Language problems were also a barrier. Often services were not convenient, so inconvenient that potential clients preferred not to use them. Finally, cost of services may have been a significant barrier. As Kimura and Browne noted, economic circumstances for Filipino families in the U.S. made things difficult; adult children often needed two jobs. Immigrant status was a particular source of economic problems affecting caregiving and ability to use services.

It may also be that social change and the setting and social arrangements in the U.S. do not present conditions that facilitate the traditional cultural approach of family care. Increased life expectancy, smaller families with fewer children and changes in women's roles including high rates of labor force participation can affect the cadre of family members available to undertake caregiver roles. Economic change that often makes it necessary for both husbands and wives to be employed in order to maintain an adequate standard of living can also limit adult children's availability. Geographic mobility, where family members spread out as they pursue their economic advantage rather than live near each other or in ethnic enclaves may also make family caregivers less available. Together these factors may conflict with traditional cultural requirements. Finally, generational differences and acculturation to U.S. society may also weaken these ties.

Ajrouch (2005) was careful to point out the tension between cultural expectations of family care—adult children's obligation to care for elderly and frail parents—and the realities of everyday life like making a living and raising children. Ajrouch conducted an extensive focus group study among Arab American elders in the Detroit metropolitan area. Respondents were Arab immigrants age 60 and older, Moslem and Christian, and included both recent immigrants and less recent immigrants. Ajrouch reported that respondents viewed nursing homes as places to avoid but they recognized that nursing homes were needed. Those with health problems were especially reluctant; their expectation was of support and care from their adult children in the event of illness and dependency. That is, their expectation was consistent with cultural beliefs. However, concern over being a burden to their children showed their ambivalence. As Ajrouch reported, while some elders were hesitant about relieving their children of their obligation to provide care, they also recognized their children's need to maintain employment and support their own households.

Radina and Barber (2004) sought to identify, systematically, factors that influenced community-based and formal services use by Hispanic caregivers. Their regression analysis identified three factors, caregiver attitude, acculturation, and family network size as predictive. Caregivers with a more positive feeling about their role, that have a larger family network, and are less acculturated to U.S. culture were *least* likely to use services. Those least positive about caregiving, more acculturated and with a smaller family network were most likely to turn to support services. These results with Hispanic adult children caregivers of elderly parents seem not inconsistent with the results reported by Kimura and Browne (2009) with Filipino caregivers.

In sum, race/ethnicity and associated cultural beliefs are a strong influence on the context and care structures of caregiving and an influence on the course of caregiving including the likelihood of turning to non-family, formal, institutional sources of care. Compared to non-Hispanic whites, ethnic minority caregivers are more likely to feel a stronger sense of family obligation and less likely to use formal care. And, compared to Anglos caregivers, ethnic minority caregivers are more likely to have social support networks to assist with caregiving.

8.1.3 Variations in the Details of Context

Material resources are usually useful in problem-solving. As previously noted (see Table 8.6) minority members generally tend to have lower incomes compared to Anglos. Specific studies of caregivers that compared non-Hispanic whites and African Americans have found African American caregivers have lower incomes and are poorer than non-Hispanic white caregivers (Horowitz and Reinhard 1995; Pinquart and Sorensen 2005; Haley et al. 2004; Sun et al. 2010; Francis et al. 2011). In studies across ethnic groups, the general finding was that ethnic minority caregivers in the U.S. also had lower socioeconomic status compared to Anglo caregivers (Pinquart and Sorensen 2005; Clark et al. 2010; Haley et al. 2004; Clay et al. 2008).

In addition to income and socioeconomic status, ethnic minority caregivers are likely to have less education compared to Anglos caregivers (Adams et al. 2002; Min and Barrio 2009; Montoro-Rodriguez and Gallagher-Thompson 2009; Herrera et al. 2008; Pinquart and Sorensen 2005). Asian Americans were not significantly different from Anglos (Pinquart and Sorensen 2005) but Mexican American caregivers had lower average education compared to African American and Anglo caregivers. African American caregivers had significantly lower average education compared to white caregivers (Adams et al. 2002).

Studies also provide generalizations that compared to Anglos, ethnic minority caregivers are:

- More likely to be younger;
- Less likely to be a spouse, more likely to be adult children of the care receiver;
- Less likely to be married;
- More likely to be female;
- More likely to be employed.

Ethnic minority caregivers generally had lower socioeconomic status, were younger and less likely to be the care receiver's spouse, more likely to be adult children compared to Anglo caregivers. When adult children are the caregivers, they are more likely to be employed (Pinquart and Sorensen 2005).

Context factors may affect patterns of care. For example, elderly African Americans are likely to be economically disadvantaged and to experience high rates of functional disability and health problems. There may also be barriers to services use such as difficulty in access, affordability, and lack of availability of services (Bullock et al. 2003). African American families are less likely to use formal services and more likely to rely on an informal caregiving network of family than non-Hispanic whites. Labor force participation by caregivers may limit time spent in providing care.

Bullock et al. (2003) interviewed a sample of elderly African American caregivers to study employed caregivers. They pointed out that African American caregivers, most often women, were employed in jobs with little time flexibility in work schedule and in jobs where they were unlikely to have sick leave or leave to care for dependents. Results showed that employed caregivers were likely to be younger than the typical caregiver. They were also younger and healthier than caregivers who were not employed. However, older caregivers provided less care, on average. Employed caregivers were likely to be an adult child rather than the care receivers' spouse, while unemployed caregivers were more likely to be a spouse or friend. Unemployed caregivers were also less likely to have alternatives to their being the caregivers; they had smaller networks and were even likely to report having no other source of help if they were not able to provide the care.

However, the researchers found that, comparing employed and not employed caregivers, the actual amount of care did not differ significantly. And, the same was true regarding the proportion of caregivers in each group who used formal services. Employed caregivers were more likely to have secondary caregivers who helped them. Still, the combination of employment and caregiving can create a demanding schedule for caregivers and contribute to their burden.

A major focus of this research of Bullock and co-workers was the relationship between caregiving and employment. The researchers reported that primary caregivers who were not employed were highly likely to have reported quitting their jobs, not seeking employment and making other job-related changes because of their caregiving responsibilities. Those not employed were more likely to report that the care receiver had no other source of help.

The researchers concluded that employed or not employed did not account for the time spent in providing care and did not account for services use among their respondents. Older caregivers who lived with the care receiver spent the most time providing care for these elderly African Americans. Socioeconomic status and the ability to purchase outside services was not a factor in formal services use. Only the level of care receivers' disability was associated with the use of services.

The condition of the care receiver, including the severity of diagnosis and severity of disability of the care receiver is an important contextual factor. In general the evidence shows that ethnic minority care receivers tend to show more severe disorders and greater disability. According to Dilworth-Anderson and Gibson (1999), blacks have a higher prevalence of dementia than other ethnic groups. Risk factors for dementia include genetic inheritance, age, head trauma, cardiovascular disease, hypertension, and diabetes. Ethnic minority elders are at greater risk of these and generally poorer health as a result of the cumulative effects over the life course of economic disadvantage and discrimination.

As shown in Tables 8.4 and 8.5, older adults from minority groups have increased levels of disability and impairments in ADLs and more physical impairments generally. African American care receivers were more physically and cognitively impaired than white care receivers. Hispanic care receivers also had more physical impairments and more behavioral problems as well (Pinquart and Sorensen 2005). Borrayo et al. (2007) added that Latinos were at higher risk of Alzheimer's disease and related dementias. Clark et al. (2010) reported that African Americans and Hispanics are at greater risk for stroke—225.2/100,000 and 166.7/100,000 respectively, compared to 136/100,000 for non-Hispanic whites. Closely related, as Clark et al. also reported, minority members also are at higher risk of hypertension, diabetes, and obesity than Anglos and African Americans and Hispanics also have lower rates of compliance with treatments and make less use of healthcare services compared to Anglos. These factors increase dementia risk.

Hilgeman et al. (2009) found that whites were more likely than African Americans to use only immediate family and were more likely to use formal services. African Americans had more members in their caregiving network which were more likely to include non-family—friends and neighbors—and more likely to share caregiving responsibilities than whites. African Americans were also less likely to use formal supports and more likely than whites to view caregiving as a natural part of the life course. African American caregivers reported lower anxiety over the caregiving role and greater religious coping and less use of psychiatric medications.

Adams et al. (2002) conducted extensive interviews over a 3 year period with spousal caregivers of dementia patients with the intent of comparing across ethnic groups. The sample included 41 Japanese Americans, 67 Anglo Americans, 49 African Americans, and 45 Mexican Americans. Spouses were both men and women though more women than men. Significant race/ethnicity effects were found for income and education of caregivers. Anglos had significantly higher incomes than the other three groups. "About $ 1,200 more per month than the Mexican- and African-American caregivers; Japanese American caregivers had about $ 700 more per month than Mexican Americans" (p. 290). Mexican American caregivers also had significantly less education (less than a high school diploma) than the other groups. African Americans averaged a high school education and Anglos averaged some college. Overall male patients were more impaired than female patients but no significant race/ethnicity effects or interaction effects were found.

Montoro-Rodriguez et al. (2009) also studied a multiethnic sample of caregivers of Alzheimer's disease patients. They found that Anglos differed from African Americans and Hispanics; caregivers were more likely to be spouses than adult children. Hispanic caregivers had less education and had been caregiving longer, a year longer on average. Anglo caregivers also had better self-reported health than African American caregivers who reported significantly better health than Hispanic caregivers. Anglos tended to have fewer caregivers than either African Americans or Hispanics. And, Hispanic patients had higher needs for help with ADLs and presented more problem behaviors compared to Anglo and African American patients.

Min and Barrio (2009) interviewed a sample of 89 Latino and 30 Anglo elders on care in the event of a hip fracture, an injury that elders are at some risk for. Authors reported that hip fractures occur 12.9/1,000 white women age 75–84 and 33.7/1,000 for those 85 or older. They also reported that Mexican American elders also have high rates approaching those of Anglo elders. In addition Anglo caregivers had significantly better self-rated health, higher educational levels, and significantly higher incomes similar to results reported by Coleman et al. (2006) and Adams et al. (2002). These findings regarding caregiver health, age, and income appear to be generally consistent across studies.

The transition to caregiving has been frequently identified as a stressful event in one's life course. The framework most often used for description has been a stress/coping model, the Stress Process Model.

8.1.4 The Stress Process Model

The stress process model recognizes the presence of stressors in people's lives. These are, "the dogged hardships, demands, conflicts, and frustrations that may be instrumental in structuring people's experiences across time and to events that may disrupt the continuities of their lives" (Pearlin et al. 1981, p. 206). Stressors may be specific life-events or more enduring, "such as having to endure economic strain, being in an exploitive job…, being drawn into a demanding caregiving role or being the target of unfair treatment because of race" (Pearlin et al. 1981, p. 206). Note that caregiving and minority status were specifically mentioned as sources of stress.

The caregiving context is made up of relationships between caregiver and care receiver and is influenced by the caregiver's age and gender and education and employment status and years of caring. The caregiving context influences objective stressors, role strain, intra-psychic strain, and outcomes. Subjective stressors affect role strain mediated by resources and coping strategies which also mediate between role strain and intra-psychic strain and between that and outcomes.

Racial and ethnic groups may vary in the perceived intensity of stressors, availability of resources, and use of coping strategies as well as the relation of stressors, resources, and strategies to caregiver outcomes. What we have called context here, is a set of factors that form the base of the caregiving situation. The context of caregiving affects the types of stressors caregivers must cope with, shapes the caregivers' duties and burden, caregivers' cognitive response to their situation (appraisal), caregivers' coping strategies and their outcomes like distress, sense of burden, depression, and declining health.

Pinquart and Sorensen (2005) developed the idea of context noting that groups may show differences on various contextual levels. For example, employment status or educational status differences may be observed at the structural or macro social level. At the interpersonal level, differences may be found in interpersonal relationships, norms of family responsibility, and extent of kinship networks. At the temporal level, differences may exist in the timing of caregiving within the life course. As we showed in the data above, situational differences among groups may exist such as the nature and severity of impairment of the person needing care. At the micro or personal level, the context may be influenced by the time management, behavioral style, coping strategies, and general health of the caregiver. Taken together, these contextual factors establish the nature of the caregivers' duties.

Duties include the extent of the caregiver's involvement with the care recipient, most often understood in terms of time commitment (e.g. hours/week). For example, the National Alliance for Caregiving (2004) reported data that in 2004 and 2009, about half of caregivers spent about 8 h per week though about 13 % said they spent more than 40 h per week.

Duties also include the various tasks the caregiver may perform. For example, help with activities of daily living (ADLs) like getting in and out of bed, getting dressed, bathing, eating, and toileting. Duties may also include help with IADLs (instrumental activities of daily living) like providing transport, help with housework, shopping, and help with managing finances and other official matters. Duties also often include advocating for recipient and mediating with agencies and professionals. Finally, duties also include just being there, watching and providing company, social contact, and support (National Alliance for Caregiving 2004). Duties may predict the burden of caregiving.

Generally, "burden" refers to costs or other consequences of the caregiver's activities. Lai (2010) described caregiver burden as the "Stress and tension and anxiety caregivers feel and experience when they are faced with problems and challenges when caring for their care receiver" (p. 200). Burden results from discomfort and strain. "Burden is a word used to describe feeling emotionally or physically heavy" (p. 201).

Biegel et al. (2007) noted that burden can be conceptualized in terms of objective burden and subjective burden. The former refers to observable events like disruptions in the everyday life of the caregiver(s) and/or family members. Subjective burden refers to emotional costs. Examples of objective costs include financial expenses, quitting or changing jobs to facilitate caregiving, disruption of family relations or social relations, or disruption of significant household routines like children's activities. The subjective dimension includes caregiver feelings of being trapped or isolated, feelings of worry, anxiety, and depressions, or negative feelings toward the person cared for (St. Onge and Lavole 1997).

Sun et al. (2010) described subjective burden as (1) caregivers' sense of being personally restricted by caregiving—not enough time for self; (2) caregivers' feeling that their health is affected; (3) caregivers concerns over monetary costs of caregiving; (4) caregivers' sense that the caregiving is not worth the effort; and (5) caregivers' irritations at the care receiver. Thus, caregiving burden is a perception of what caregiving means to the caregiver, a kind of appraisal of the activity.

Duties and burdens as well as contextual factors like the lack of resources and the severity of the care receiver's disability are potential stressors, sources of stress for the caregiver(s). Stress in turn can have consequences for the health and well-being of the caregiver. However these consequences can be mediated by the caregiver's cognitive appraisal of the burden. Appraisal refers to the meaning the caregiver assigns to their activities and the consequences of their activities. A more positive appraisal may result in less distress. In addition, the presence of social support and assistance and the caregiver's coping strategies may also serve to help with stress management and reduction which can mediate the onset of distress and negative health consequences for the caregiver.

The context and duties together influence the incidence of stressors, events or processes that require caregivers to make adaptations. An example might be helping the care receiver get dressed which can be easy if they are easy to deal with and have awareness and the physical agility to put their own clothes on. The task can become more stressful if the person is cranky, oppositional, easily threatened, and/or lacks the motor ability to perform the task or assist the caregiver. But potentially stressful situations become less stressful if the caregiver has a positive appraisal of their task. For example, one caregiver might become quite stressed trying to help her mother get dressed. Another may have the sense of loyalty, affection, and compassion for her mother and is able to make light of the hassle while helping her mother get dressed. The objective events may be similar but the caregiver's cognitive interpretations are significantly different.

The combination of the objective stressor and the subjective appraisal create the extent of stress that the caregiver might feel. Stress can be reduced depending on the extent of social support they receive in carrying out their duties. Stress can also be reduced depending on the coping skills that the caregiver has. Over time, continued stress can result in negative consequences for caregivers' health, mental health, or general sense of well-being. However, these can be held in check by more positive appraisals, by the presence of social support, and by effective coping skills. Figure 8.1 presents the above graphically. The remainder of this chapter will review ethnic variations in caregiving by factors of this adaptation of the stress process model. Note that research on racial and ethnic variations in caregiving often compares minorities to white Anglos.

The transition to caregiving has been identified as a stressful event in one's life course. And caregiving for a spouse or other family member with a diagnosis of Alzheimer's disease or a related dementia can be particularly stressful. The following expression summarizes the views of many commentators:

> Caring for a loved one with Alzheimer's disease or a related disorder (ADRD) can have a devastating effect on the emotional and physical well-being of the primary caregiver. (Hilgeman et al. 2009, p. 248)

Among the sources of stress, caregivers daily bear witness to the progressive deterioration of their loved ones, their husband or wife, mother, father, or other family members, as the caregiver compares them to the person they once were. A particular source of stress with dementia is often the lack of understanding and an absence of information on the part of caregivers. Hinton et al. (2005) asserted that older people and families from ethnic minorities are likely to be less familiar with the medical model of dementia and have a less clear understanding of dementia than Anglos. They conducted qualitative studies among Anglos, African-Americans, Asian-Americans (Chinese and Vietnamese), and Latinos to determine each group's

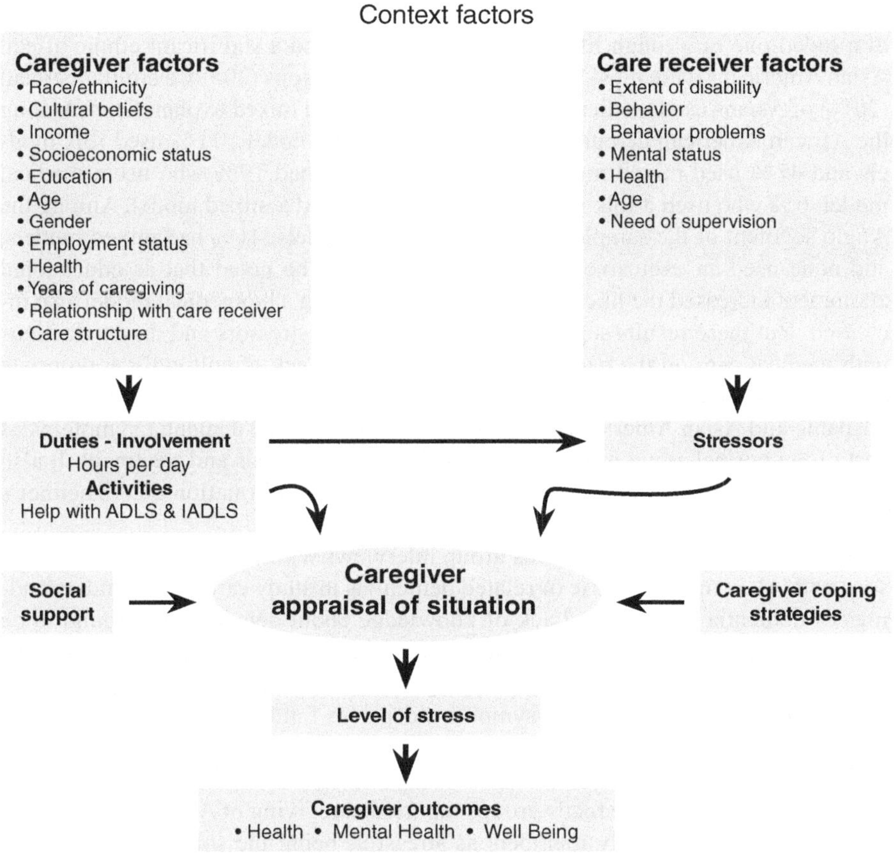

Fig. 8.1 Schematic diagram of stress process model

explanatory models of dementia and patterns of help seeking. Participants (n = 92) were all primary caregivers for an older family member with a dementia diagnosis. Most often they were daughters living with their parent. Overall 64 % of participants were adult children, 26 % were spouses, 80 % were female, 70 % lived with the care receivers. Each participant was interviewed in their native language.

Results were that 36 % used biomedical explanations and referred to disease or disorder. They made attributions to brain pathology including neurotransmitters. They also referred to health factors like smoking, overweight, and other vascular risk factors reflecting a medical model. Ten percent of respondents used folk models to explain dementia. Folk models explain dementia as either the normal effect of aging or the result of psychological stress with dementia as a mental illness. At least one respondent mentioned spirit possession.

The remainder, 54 %, used explanations that mixed folk models and a medical model. For example, the caregiver might use the medical labels, Alzheimer's disease, but explain it as a result of worry or loneliness or stress such as the loss of a loved one or a tough life. The breakdown showed a significant ethnic affect. Asian Americans were most likely to use folk explanations (20 %); a similar percent (20 %) of Asians used medical explanations, 60 % used mixed explanations. Among the African American caregivers, 42 % used medical models, 11 % used folk models and 47 % used mixed models. Latino caregivers had 19 % who use a medical model, 6 % who used a folk model, and 75 % who used a mixed model. Among the Anglo segment of the sample 59 % used medical models, 41 % had mixed models, and none used an exclusively folk model. It should be noted that as educational attainment increased the likelihood of a caregiver using a biomedical model also increased. But these results suggest possible sources of stressors and dissatisfactions with medical care on the part of some caregivers or lack of culturally appropriate approaches to treatment by providers. Or as Levkoff et al. (1999) suggested, some Hispanic and Asian American caregivers' interpretations of dementia symptoms as part of the normal aging process may delay timely diagnosis and treatment. It also suggests less than thorough diffusion of public health information on Alzheimer's and related dementias.

Borrayo et al. (2007) used focus group interviews with Latino caregivers of persons with Alzheimer's disease or related dementias to study caregivers' understandings of dementia caregiving. Lack of knowledge about dementia was found to be a deterrent to recognition of symptoms. Latinos with little education may view dementia, incorrectly, as part of normal aging or as a mental illness caused by nerves or the evil eye. Not recognizing symptoms deprives Latino caregivers of information that might be useful in their coping with caregiving and the course of illness of their care receiver.

The respondents of the focus groups reported caregiving of Alzheimer's disease or related dementia family members as stressful; being the sole caregiver led to the most hardship; observations of the person's decline and their inability to do anything about it caused the caregivers to experience grief and sadness. They also reported having little information initially and being overwhelmed by the responsibilities and having no time for themselves with the demanding schedule needs of the care receiver. Some had to quit jobs. The respondents also reported a variety of coping strategies. Some were active coping; changing one's schedule to meet caregiving demands, avoiding argument with the care receiver by acquiescing, information seeking regarding dementia and services, and seeking social support when available. Cognitive coping strategies included taking a problem solving, solution-focused approach to challenges, self-talk, developing effective communication strategies for communicating with the care receiver, and acceptance. Spiritual strategies included relying on God and spirituality for gaining emotional and spiritual strength to deal with the challenges associated with caregiving.

Coping styles or coping strategies are often categorized as either *active coping or emotion focused coping.* The former refers to steps such as seeking social support, problem solving, information seeking, or planning and enacting change. Emotion focused includes denial or escape or avoidance. Religious coping is another approach.

Montoro-Rodriguez and Gallegher-Thompson (2009) were among many investigators that noted that caregivers of persons diagnosed with dementia have an increased risk of burden, stress and depression. Their general orientation was consistent with the stress process model but they tested models to see if model factors, such as coping and appraisals such as self-efficacy varied by culture—specifically between Latinas and Anglo women who were caregivers of persons with diagnoses of Alzheimer's disease or related dementias.

Their sample included 89 Hispanic and 96 Anglo women, family caregivers, a mixture of spouses and adult children. There were more daughters among the Latinas and more spouses among the Anglo women. Also, Latina caregivers had less education, lower income, and lower health ratings, were more likely to be employed and provided more hours of care per day.

Measures of coping showed significant ethnic difference. Latinas used fewer active coping strategies like seeking social support, and used more escape/avoidance coping compared to the Anglo caregivers. Ethnic differences in appraisals were also found; Latinas showed higher self-efficacy appraisal and lower level of perceived burden. Analysis also showed that Latina caregivers' lower level of burden was associated with their ability to control upsetting thoughts and through the use of avoidance coping strategies.

Gerdner et al. (2007) conducted an ethnographic study of African American caregivers in a rural Southern setting, the Arkansas delta region. These caregivers provided care for family members with what was locally called chronic confusion. The key for these caregivers was their spirituality, their religious beliefs and practices and their faith in God; "prayer was the most commonly used coping strategy" (p. 369). As Gerdner et al. reported, "Prayer is viewed by African American persons as a means of communicating with God in much the same way one would communicate with a friend or family member" (p. 369). Some of the respondents identified God as "their primary source of emotional support" or reported "Praying 'lifts my burdens.'"

Jones-Cannon and Davis (2005) studied coping among African American daughters using focus groups and semi-structured interviews. Most participants reported that religion, faith, and prayer helped them cope. "They felt that their faith in God and Scripture had been instrumental in enabling them to cope with caregiving" (p. 121). The participants also reported that social support helped, that the support of friends and family and a good parent-child relationship were essential for coping. A few mentioned respite care by a person paid to be there. Others mentioned caregiver support group sessions as very helpful.

Other coping strategies included reduction of expectations, making positive comparisons and construction of a larger sense of illness that helped them to accept their parents as they were. Reducing future orientation also helped. So did information seeking; making sense of their parent's dementia helped with knowing what to expect which helped with coping. But most rated themselves as very religious and often prayed for strength.

Religion, prayer, and faith in God were instrumental in helping African American daughters cope with caregiving. Spirituality was a theme that predominated throughout focus group discussions. It was the belief by many that without prayer and God, they would not have had the strength to continue their caregiver role (Jones-Cannon and Davis 2009, p. 122).

Caregiving was a commitment to the Scriptural Commandment to honor thy father and mother.

Herrera et al. (2009) questioned whether religiosity or religious coping eased Mexican American family caregivers' feelings. Religiosity included (1) "organizational religiosity," the public aspect of belonging to and attendance at a religious organization; (2) "non-organizational religiosity," the private practice of religious rituals; and (3) intrinsic religiosity, one's internal beliefs. Results showed that Latino caregivers with greater organizational and intrinsic religiosity were less likely to perceive burden associated with caregiving. Caregivers with greater non-organizational religiosity were more likely to have less well-being and greater sense of burden. Non-organizational religiosity—private prayer, Bible study, and meditation on their own—was not associated with the social support that institutional attendance and worship provide.

Morano and King (2005) hypothesized that religion would be a coping resource; specifically they hypothesized that among caregivers increasing religiosity would be associated with decreasing depression and increasing self-acceptance. Morano and King had a sample composed of 348 African American, Hispanic, and Anglo caregivers who responded to their questionnaire. Respondents were primarily women (75 %) about half spousal caregivers, half caring for a parent. Results included an ethnicity effect for religiosity. African Americans scored higher than the others, Anglos the lowest. Religiosity was related to lower depression and to greater self-acceptance.

Some stressors are associated with the care receivers' objective disabilities. Problem behaviors of persons with dementia, and caretaking activities like help with daily activities particularly add to the stressors. The stress process model asserts that stressors—life events or ongoing problems (Pearlin et al. 1981, p. 338) are sources of stress for individuals. Contextual conditions can influence the extent of stress experienced by caregivers. Context features such as caregivers' own health, and care receivers' disability and behaviors, hours of care provided as well as issues of employment, child care, family conflict and availability of resources and funds are all potential stressors.

Stress has consequences affecting the health and/or mental health of individuals exposed to stress. But these outcomes are not necessarily inevitable. Stressors, events or situations that require individuals to adapt to change, are inevitable, but individuals' cognitive response to stressors, the availability of resources, social supports, and coping strategies also can affect the outcome.

Adams et al. (2002) used structured interviews with spousal caregivers currently residing with their wife or husband who had a dementia diagnosis. The research, conducted in California, included samples of Japanese-American caregivers (n=41), African American caregivers (n=49), Mexican American caregivers (n=45), and Anglo American caregivers (n=67). Caregivers' appraisal, coping styles, and social support were among the issues studied along with characteristics of the care receiver and caregiver outcomes.

Caregivers' cognitive response to caregiving, their appraisal, affects consequences for caregivers. Adams et al. (2002) described six dimensions of appraisal, three positive and three negative. Positive appraisal appears to be a global evaluation of caregiving. Self efficacy appraisal appears to be one's evaluation of their personal ability to handle caregiving. Spiritual appraisal seems to relate to feelings about a spiritual purpose to one's caregiving. Pessimistic appraisal is associated with a gloomy outlook. And lack of support appraisal is associated with thoughts about getting help from others.

Research showed significant ethnic effects on each of these factors. Mexican Americans scored higher than Anglos on most appraisal categories, positive appraisals and pessimistic appraisals as well as spiritual appraisals and perceived lack of social support appraisals. Authors interpreted this result in terms of the cultural value of family responsibility for care provides a source for positive appraisal. But the expectation of high levels of social support that does not actually occur promotes pessimism.

African Americans also showed higher positive appraisal and spiritual appraisal compared to Anglos. Otherwise African American and Anglo appraisals were similar. Mexican Americans and African Americans were similar on spiritual appraisal though Mexican Americans scored highest on pessimistic appraisals and were more likely to regard their situation pessimistically.

Adams et al. also compared groups on coping styles and resources for coping. The strategies a person uses for coping are associated with their approach to the situation they have to cope with. Positive coping strategies include information seeking, problem solving, and obtaining social support. Avoidance and denial are other, less effective, coping styles. Reframing, reappraisal, changing the definition of the situation is somewhere in between these two. Religious involvement is another coping strategy as worshipers seek comfort and stress reduction through their faith and through prayer. Resources for coping include social support and social networks including extended family.

Data showed significant ethnic and gender effects for escape/avoidance coping and seeking social support, but not for the positive strategies. Mexican American caregivers scored higher on escape/avoidance coping compared to Anglos and African Americans. Japanese Americans scored higher on seeking social support than Anglos. As for resources, African Americans had significantly greater levels of social support than the other three groups and Japanese Americans were significantly lower on religiosity. Anglos, Latinos and African Americans were similar in their use of religion as a coping resource. Age, income, and education did not affect or alter these results (Adams et al. 2002, p. 293).

Adams et al. found that Anglos had significantly higher incomes than the other three groups and higher education than African-Americans and Mexican Americans. Mexican Americans showed the longest average duration of caregiving. Outcome measures were general psychiatric symptoms/distress (measured by SCL—90, a checklist of 90 symptoms, each rated by extent of distress) and a mood questionnaire (Older Adult Health and Mood Questionnaire) that assesses extent of depressive symptoms.

The depression outcome measures showed significant ethnic and gender effects. Mexican American dementia caregivers in this sample had higher depressive symptom levels than Anglo and African American caregivers. Specifically, Adams et al. reported:

...that 89 % of the Mexican American caregivers reported clinically significant depressive symptoms (51 % of whom had probable major depression...). This compared to the Anglo American rate of 66 % and African American caregiver rate of 57 % (Adams et al. 2002, p. 290).

The authors added that 27 % of the Japanese Americans were also probable for major depression.

The general psychiatric distress measures did not show a significant ethnic effect but there was a trend showing Mexican American and Japanese American caregivers were more distressed than Anglos and African American caregivers.

Haley et al. (2004) tested hypotheses about African American and non-Hispanic white family caregivers of persons with dementia. In earlier research, Haley and his colleagues had compared African American caregivers with non-Hispanic white dementia caregivers. They found that both African American caregivers and non-caregivers had poorer self reported health compared to whites (Haley et al. 1995). With regard to appraisals, they also found that African American dementia caregivers were less upset, had more positive appraisal of caregiving stressors and higher self efficacy appraisal than their white counterparts (Haley et al. 1996). These prior results prompted Haley et al. (2004) to hypothesize that African American dementia caregivers would show less psychological distress, more positive appraisal, less distress, and more subjective benefit from caregiving compared to comparable whites. They also hypothesized that African Americans would show poorer health and more unhealthy behaviors and higher levels of religious behaviors than whites (Haley et al. 2004, p. 18).

Data for this study came from 720 primary caregivers from the REACH program: Resources for Enhancing Alzheimer's Caregivers' Health, "a multi-site, multi-year intervention program of support for dementia caregivers." At the time of this study, according to the authors, it was, "one of the largest studies to date" comparing whites and African American family caregivers of persons with dementia from diverse regions of the United States. Comparisons of coping resources showed a significant ethnic effect across all sites with no ethnic by site interaction. Compared to Anglos, African American caregivers were significantly more likely to report frequent prayer, frequent religious attendance, and rate religion as "very important."

In general results confirmed the hypotheses. African American caregivers showed better well-being, less psychological distress, lower depression, and lower anxiety scores. In addition, African American appraisals of potential stressors were found to be "more benign." African Americans were less distressed by memory and behavior problems of their care receivers. African Americans also showed significantly better appraisals of caregiving in general. No significant ethnic effects were found for physical health. It may be the case that more positive appraisals are a factor in African Americans' having less depression and less psychological distress from caregiving.

Hilgeman et al. (2009) tested the stress process model with an ethnically diverse sample of caregivers of persons with dementia diagnoses (ADRD) using data from the REACH II project. The sample of 642 caregivers included about one-third each of white, African-American, and Hispanic caregivers (34.8, 33, and 32.2 % respectively). The model proposed that context factors help define stressors that caregivers face, their appraisal of the stressors and the health and/or mental health and well-being outcomes for caregivers. Context variables included in this study were caregiver age, gender, education, employment status, relation to care receiver, and years of caregiving. They also included the nature and extent of the care receiver's disability.

Stressors include both objective stressors and subjective stressors. Objective stressors are mental status and problem behaviors of the care receiver, and extent of the care receivers need for assistance and amount of assistance provided for ADLs and IADLs. Subjective stressors are caregivers' cognitive responses to problem behaviors, to specific caring activities, and to caregiving itself—appraisals. Context and stressors influence feelings related to maintaining multiple roles, role strain, which includes work related and income producing roles. Intra-psychic strain is also influenced; one's sense of self and self efficacy, one's confidence in their caregiving and ability to cope with the challenges. All of these influence health and well-being outcomes but may be mediated by social support and coping skills.

Results reported by Hilgeman et al. (2009) showed significant ethnic effects for objective and subjective stress, role strain, intra-psychic strain, resources, and caregiver outcomes. African Americans showed less objective stress than Hispanics and Anglos and less subjective stress than Anglos though greater subjective stress than Hispanics. Hispanics showed the highest objective stress and the least subjective stress. Anglos also showed higher intra-psychic strain than either African Americans or Hispanics (Hilgeman et al. 2009, p. 255; Table 2). African American caregivers also had significantly more role strain than Anglo or Hispanic caregivers. The effect of role strain was greater for caregivers with few resources (p. 257). Analysis also showed significant ethnic and gender effects for intra-psychic strain. "Specifically, more role strain, fewer resources, being female, being a spouse, and more education were related to higher levels of intra-psychic strain." (p. 257) Anglos had higher intra-psychic strain than African Americans or Latinos.

Stevens et al. (2004) sought to compare racial differences in nursing home placement of persons with dementia. They noted that persons diagnosed with dementia (ADRD) are at high risk for nursing home placement, probably because of their functional limitations and problem behaviors that can be significantly stressful for family caregivers. Caregivers' appraisal of caregiving and caregivers' burden as well as care receivers' health may also be predictive. In particular, this research investigated whether racial differences in appraisals, coping, social support, and caregiver depression were related to nursing home placement. Data came from 215 caregiver/care receiver dyads.

Results showed that nursing home placement rates were significantly lower for African American caregivers over time. Results also showed significant ethnic effects on two measures of stressfulness appraisals: caregiver appraisals of stressfulness of memory and stressfulness of behavior problems of care receiver. White caregivers showed significantly higher stress responses, significantly higher avoidance coping, and significantly higher depression compared to African American caregivers. Stevens et al. reported that, "white care recipients with dementia were placed nearly 2.5 times the rate at which African American care recipients were placed" (p. 388).

Stevens et al. also reported that higher SES and older care receiver age were predictive of a shorter time to placement. In addition, caregiver stressfulness appraisal of care receiver's memory and behavior problems and self care impairment also led to an earlier placement rate than caregivers who had a more benign appraisal of these issues. White caregivers also placed their dementia care receivers significantly sooner in the course of illness and caregiving than did African American caregivers. In addition to ethnicity, higher SES and care receiver age and non-spousal caregiver were also associated with earlier placement.

Ethnic differences in placement were interpreted as related to differences in cultural orientations to caregiving. It is likely that cultural norms and strong expectations of family caregiving among African Americans played a part. In addition, cultural-historical issues such as African American distrust of formal healthcare systems may also contribute to the lower rate of placement by African American caregivers.

8.2 Summary

Our premise here has been that caregiving is related to the ethnic and cultural context in which the caregiving takes place. The evidence seems to support ethnic variations in care structures, appraisals of caregiving, and coping strategies. One theme that emerged from our brief review is the preference among Hispanics, Asian Americans, and African Americans for family caregiving over formal services and institutional care. Along with this we learn that these ethnic groups often were unaware of the existence of services or did not know how to access them. In addition, ethnic group members often found services providers and services discriminatory, disrespectful, and culturally insensitive. Additional barriers to use of services often included language barriers, inconvenient hours, problems of accessibility, cost, and availability of staff. Lai (2010) pointed out:

> Policy makers should consider the limitations and challenges faced by individual family caregivers and should not take filial piety or obligations for granted. Without adequate support and tangible resources, the "good will" of family caregivers will eventually burn out. (Lai 2010, p. 217)

Culturally sensitive services, including language where appropriate, can and should be available. In addition, health education programs and caregiver support groups can help reduce caregiver strain. It was reported that a stress reduction program for Chinese dementia caregivers improve participants' feelings and appraisals about caregiving and improved caregivers' quality of life compared to a comparison group that received telephone support. Learning coping skills in dealing with dementia was beneficial to these caregivers.

Sun et al. (2010) also called attention to services for rural dementia caregivers, a group they called "Largely invisible to health and social services providers" (p. 300). Though many caregivers become isolated, Sun and colleagues remarked, "These [rural] caregivers often undertake significant responsibility for the care of their relatives, often in isolation and without prior training in performing caregiving tasks" (p. 300).

The evidence also suggests that faith-based organizations, local or neighborhood religious centers (churches, synagogues, mosques, etc.) may be culturally appropriate ways to reach people with information and case finding as well as locations for caregiver support groups. As Sun and colleagues pointed out, church-based health promotion programs have been found to be effective.

As the United States continues on its course toward increasing ethnic diversity and toward advancing age and increased likelihood of disability, the development of culturally appropriate and culturally sensitive services and service providers will be essential to meeting public health needs.

8.3 Questions for Discussion

1. What are some generalizations about ethnic minority caregivers that distinguish them from nonminority caregivers?
2. Explain the differences between "objective burden" and "subjective burden" in caregiving.
3. Explain the Stress Process Model.
4. What are some reasons ethnic minorities distrust formal healthcare services and use them less than Anglos?
5. Explain marianismo in Mexican-American culture.

References

Adams, B., Aranda, M. P., Kemp, B., & Takagi, K. (2002). Ethnic and gender differences in distress among Anglo American, African American, Japanese American and Mexican American spousal caregivers of persons with dementia. *Journal of Clinical Geropsychology, 8*(4), 279–301.

Ajrouch, K. J. (2005). Arab-American immigrant elders' views about social support. *Aging and Society, 25,* 655–673.

Biegel, D. E., Ishler, K., Katz, S. & Johnson, P. (2007). Predictors of burden of family caregivers of women with substance use disorders or co-occurring substance and mental disorders. *Journal of social work practice in the addictions.* 7(1/2) 2007.

Borrayo, E. A., Goldwaser, G., Vacha-Haase, T., & Hepburn, K. W. (2007). An inquiry into Latino caregivers' experience caring for older adults with Alzheimer's disease and related dementias. *Journal of Applied Gerontology, 26*(5), 486–505.

Bullock, K., Crawford, S. L., & Tennstedt, S. L. (2003). Employment and caregiving: Exploration of African American caregivers. *Social Work, 48*(2), 150–162.
Clark, A. N., Sander, A. M., Pappados, M. R., Evans, G. L., Truchen, M. A., & Choi-Tan, F. Y. (2010). Caregiver characteristics and their relationship to health service utilization in minority patients with first episode stroke. *NeuroRehabilitation, 27,* 95–104.
Clay, O. J., Roth, D. L., Wadley, V. G., & Haley, W. E. (2008). Changes in social support and their impact on psychosocial outcome over a five year period for African American and white dementia caregivers. *International Journal of Geriatric Psychiatry, 23,* 857–862.
Coleman, M., Ganong, L. H., & Rothrauff, T. C. (2006). Racial and ethnic similarities and differences in beliefs about intergenerational assistance to older adults after divorce and remarriage. *Family Relations, 55,* 576–587.
Dilworth-Anderson, P., & Gibson, B. E. (1999). Ethnic minority perspectives on dementia, caregiving, and interventions. *Generations, 23*(Fall), 40–45.
Francis, L. E., Bowman, K. F., Kypriotakis, G., & Rose, J. H. (2011). Relationships and emotional well-being among African-American and white advanced cancer caregivers. *Patient Education and Counseling, 85,* 446–453.
Gerdner, L. A., Tripp-Reimer, T., & Simpson, H. C. (2007). Hard lives, God's help, and struggling through: Caregiving in Arkansas Delta. *Journal of Cross Cultural Gerontology, 22,* 355–374.
Haley, W. E., West, C. A., Wadley, V. G., Ford, G. R., White, F. A., & Barrett, J. J., et al. (1995). Psychological, social, and health impact of caregiving: A comparison of black and white dementia caregivers and non-caregivers. *Psychology and Aging, 10,* 540–552.
Haley, W. E., Roth, D., Coleton, M., Ford, G. R., West, C. A., Collins, R. P., & Isobe, T. L. (1996). Appraisal, coping, and social support as mediators of well-being in black and white family caregivers of patients with Alzheimer's disease. *Journal of Consulting and Clinical Psychology, 64,* 121–129.
Haley, W. E., Gitlin, L. N., Wisniewski, S. R, Mahoney, D. F., Coon, D. W., Winter, L., Corcoran, M., Schinfeld, S., & Ory, M. (2004). Well-being, appraisal, and coping in African American and Caucasian dementia caregivers: Findings from the REACH study. *Aging and Mental Health, 8*(4), 316–329.
Herrera, A. P., Lee, J., Palos, G., & Torres-Vigil, I. (2008). Cultural influences in the patterns of long term care use among Mexican American family caregivers. *Journal of Applied Gerontology, 27*(2), 141–165.
Herrera, A. P., Lee, J. W., Nanyonjo, R. D., Laufman, L. E., & Torres-Vigil, I. (2009). Religious coping and caregiver well-being in Mexican-American families. *Aging and Mental Health, 13*(1), 84–91.
Hilgeman, M. M., Durkin, D. W., Sun, F., DeCoster, J., Allen, R. S., Gallagher-Thompson, D., & Burgio, L. D. (2009). Testing a theoretical model of the stress process in Alzheimer's caregivers with race as a moderator. *The Gerontologist, 49*(2), 248–261.
Hinojosa, M. S., Zsembik, B., & Rittman, M. (2009). Patterns of informal care among Puerto Rican, African American, and white stroke survivors. *Ethnicity and Health, 14*(6), 591–606.
Hinton, L., Franz, C. E., Yeo, G., & Levkoff, S. (2005). Conceptions of dementia in a multiethnic sample of family caregivers. *Journal of the American Geriatric Society, 53,* 1405–1410.
Horowitz, A. V., & Reinhard, S. C. (1995). Ethnic differences in caregiving duties and burdens among parents and siblings of persons with severe mental illnesses. *Journal of Health and Social Behavior, 36*(2), 138–150.
Jones-Cannon, S., & Davis, B. L. (2005). Coping among African American daughters caring for aging parents. *The ABNF Journal, 16,* 118–123.
Kimura, J., & Browne, C. V. (2009). Eldercare in a Filipino community: Older women's attitudes toward caregiving and service use. *Journal of Women and Aging, 21,* 229–243.
Lai, D. W. L. (2010). Filial piety, caregiving appraisal and caregiving burden. *Research on Aging, 32*(2), 200–223.
Lee, Y., & Bronstein, L. R. (2010). When do Korean American dementia caregivers find meaning in caregiving?: The role of culture and differences between spouse and child caregivers. *Journal of Ethnic and Cultural Diversity in Social Work, 19,* 73–86.

Levkoff, S., Levy, B., & Weitzman, P. F. (1999). The role of religion and ethnicity in the help seeking of family caregivers of elders with Alzheimer's disease and related disorders. *Journal of Cross Cultural Gerontology, 14,* 335–356.

Marks, N. F., Lambert, J. D., Jun, H., & Song, J. (2008). Psychosocial moderators of the effects of transitioning into filial caregiving on mental and physical health. *Research on Aging, 30*(3), 358–389.

Min, J. W., & Barrio, C. (2009). Cultural values and caregiver preference for Mexican American and non-Latino white elders. *Journal of Cross Cultural Gerontology, 24,* 225–239.

Montoro-Rodriguez, J., & Gallagher-Thompson, D. (2009). The role of resources and appraisals in predicting burden among Latina and non-Hispanic white female caregivers: A cast of an expanded socio-cultural model of stress and coping. *Aging and Mental Health, 13*(5), 648–658.

Morano, C. L., & King, D. (2005). Religiosity as a mediator of caregiver well-being: Does ethnicity make a difference? *Journal of Gerontological Social Work, 45,* 69–84.

National Alliance for Caregiving and AARP. (1 April 2004). Caregiving in the U.S. *AARP.*

National Center for Health Statistics. (2012). *Health United States: Trend tables.* Hyattsville: National Center for Health Statistics.

Pearlin, L. I., Lieberman, M. A., Menaghan, E. G., & Mullan, J. T. (1981). The stress process. *Journal of Health and Social Behavior, 22*(4), 337–356.

Pinquart, M., & Sorensen, S. (2005). Ethnic differences in stressors, resources, and psychological outcomes of family caregiving: A meta-analysis. *The Gerontologist, 45*(1), 90–106.

Radina, M. E., & Barber, C. E. (2004). Utilization of formal support services among Hispanic Americans caring for aging parents. *Journal of Gerontological Social Work, 43*(2/3), 5–23.

Radina, M. E., Gibbons, H. M., & Lim, J. Y. (2009). Explicit versus implicit family decision making strategies among Mexican American caregiving adult children. *Marriage and Family Review, 45,* 392–411.

St. Onge, M., & Lavole, F. (1997). The experience of caregiving among mothers of adults suffering from psychotic disorders: Factors associated with their psychological distress. *American Journal of Community Psychology, 25,* 73–94.

Stevens, A., Owen, J., Roth, D., Clay, O., Bartolucci, A., & Haley, W. (2004). Predictors of time to nursing home placement in white and African American individuals with dementia. *Journal of Aging and Health, 16*(3), 375–397.

Sun, F., Kosberg, J. I., Leeper, J., Kaufman, A. V., & Burgio, L. (2010). Racial differences in perceived burden of rural dementia caregivers: The mediating effect of religiosity. *Journal of Applied Gerontology, 29*(2), 290–307.

U.S. Census Bureau. (2012a). *American fact finder.* Washington: U.S. Census Bureau.

U.S. Census Bureau. (2013). *Statistical abstract of the United States 2012.* Washington: U.S. Census Bureau. (National Center for Health Statistics (2012).

Weng, S., & Nguyen, P. V. (2011). Factors affecting elder caregiving in multigenerational Asian American families. *Families in Society, 92*(3), 329–335.

Chapter 9
Outsourced and Specialized Caregiving

9.1 Introduction

Hochschild (2012) has described how, over the past century, slowly, but persistently, the market has come to dominate American life. Many aspects of American life have slipped from the realms of community, commons, and government into the market. Work and personal services have become more specialized, more technologically-oriented, and more tailored to meet individual needs. We have outsourced ourselves to the degree that every stage of life has a corresponding market service, even death.

While it is difficult to consider hired caregivers to be part of the family, formal work contracts are now common ways to assure that aging, disabled and dying loved ones will be protected, cared for, and loved. Hochschild stated, "The most profound personal experiences may become something we purchase—especially when customs linking us to generations past have lost their meaning" (p. 178). "We try to adapt to the market way of life and protect ourselves from its potentially depersonalizing effects by not depersonalizing our bonds with others to make the market feel less like a market" (p. 224).

This chapter explores how the need for long distance caregiving is substantial and growing, and how the provision of care from a distance has contributed to the growth of specialized caregiving. As people live longer lives and acquire disabling chronic illnesses with complex needs, it becomes necessary to provide a greater range of specialized services to meet those needs.

9.2 Caring from a Distance

Caregivers who live apart from their care recipients face special challenges of managing care from a distance, often including travel to another city, state or country, into their already busy lives at home and work. The spatial separation of family members, although not a prerequisite for maintaining close family ties, is an important issue in how caregivers deal with family responsibilities. The provision of care

J. G. Bruhn, H. M. Rebach, *The Sociology of Caregiving*,
Clinical Sociology: Research and Practice, DOI 10.1007/978-94-017-8857-1_9,

from a distance can reduce the frequency of visiting and informal assistance with certain activities and support tasks that are not feasible when family members live far away (Bledsoe et al. 2010).

Distance matters because of the possibility of the reduced availability of care for elders and the disabled and the physical, emotional, and the financial toll placed on family caregivers who must travel to the care recipient(s). The challenges can be particularly great for carers who do not have close relationships with the care recipient, or those carers who have multiple caregiving responsibilities such as caring for both children and aging parents (Neal et al. 2008). Unfortunately there are families who live in the same city as their institutionalized relative and visit them only on special holidays. Often the family chooses to outsource total care to a formal caregiver, especially as the family experiences conflicting family-care role responsibilities such as schedule flexibility, time off of work, or have become exhausted.

9.2.1 Long Distance Defined

The National Council on Aging has defined long-distance caregiving as those carers who "live 1 h or more away" from the care recipient. Research has shown that distance plays an important role in family decision-making about who will do the caregiving.[1] Usually the nearest sibling takes on the major responsibility regardless of work obligations, but many caregivers receive help from family, friends, and neighbors (MetLife Mature Market Institute 2004).

9.2.2 Long-Distance Caregiving

The distance between the care recipient's place of residence and that of the caregiver has a major effect on the type and frequency of care. Because of geographical mobility family caregivers often live in different cities or even regions than their care recipients. Indeed, according to the 2010 U.S. Census about 16 % of Americans move each year. Long-distance caregiving has been increasing over the past decade. A MetLife study found that at least 5 million caregivers live 1 h or more away from the person for whom they care (MetLife Mature Market Institute 2004). Most long-distance caregivers share responsibilities with siblings or paid caregivers or both. Most elders want to live in their own homes, for some this is possible with safety renovations. However, not all care recipients are homeowners or can afford renovations. Some care recipients move to retirement communities that provide different living units for residents with differing abilities. Yet, some units are expensive to buy, monthly maintenance fees are expensive, making this option unaffordable. A small number of care recipients live in rehabilitation centers for short-terms. Between 5 and 6 % of care recipients live in a long-term facility, or nursing or group home with caregivers making regular or periodic visits to monitor the care being provided.

[1] See Moore et al. (2001).

When family members cannot provide care, especially if they are employed full-time, and a long-distance caregiver, and there are no other family living nearby, they may have to outsource their family member's care.

Long-distance caregivers face unique difficulties (Koerin and Harrigan 2003). Long-distance caregiving creates challenges in assessing the needs of the care recipient which change. While critical events such as falls or illness provide obvious indicators of need, many older adults experience gradual subtle declines in functioning that may need medical attention. Once the need for assistance has been identified, locating services and monitoring them is a challenge particularly in rural areas or small towns where fewer services exist. Given the complexities of care created by change and aging some caregivers hire a geriatric care manager, who is frequently a social worker, to assess, monitor, and coordinate services.

Coordination and follow through are time consuming and complex enough when the family decision-maker is geographically separated from the care recipient, but family relationships may become further strained because of the costs of time, travel, and emotional burdens of guilt when they feel that they are not as available as they wish they could be (Bookman and Kimbrel 2011). Outsourcing daily care can help, but emotions cannot be outsourced.

As Neal et al. (2008) have written, "There are many long-distance caregivers who ultimately choose to eliminate the boundaries associated with distance by moving their family member closer, moving themselves closer to the care recipient, taking a leave of absence from work, or leaving their job entirely" (pp. 116–117).

9.2.3 Long-Distance Care of a Family Member with Dementia

In 2009, an estimated 10.9 million family members and friends provided unpaid care for a person with Alzheimer's disease or other dementia. Many people with Alzheimer's or other dementias also have other serious medical conditions such as heart disease, cancer, and diabetes. Their family caregiver and other unpaid caregivers try to manage these conditions in addition to the dementia. Nine percent of the 10.9 million family and other unpaid caregivers of people with Alzheimer's and other dementias live more than 2 h from the person for whom they provide care and another 6 % live 1–2 h away. Family caregivers of people with dementia are more likely than caregivers of older people to assist in three or more activities of daily living (ADLs) compared to caregivers of older people, and to arrange and supervise services from an agency. Because Alzheimer's and other dementias develop slowly, most caregivers spend many years in the caregiving role. At any point 32 % of family members have been caregivers for 5 years or longer. More than 40 % of family caregivers rate the emotional stress as high and as many as one-third experience depression. Long-distance caregivers of Alzheimer's patients had higher out-of-pocket expenditures compared to other caregivers. People with Alzheimer's and other dementias are high users of healthcare, long-term and hospice care. Based on average per person payments from all sources of healthcare and long-term care for people age 65 and older with dementias total payments for 2010 for Medicare and Medicaid are expected to be $ 172 billion (Alzheimer's Association 2010).[2]

Dementias test the boundaries between home and work life. The slow but steady progression of dementia eventually makes it impossible for family caregivers to balance or juggle work and home life. Some or all of the care of dementia patients needs to be outsourced. While each culture will need to address its consequences, there is a growing worldwide epidemic currently that presents severe challenges to caregiving (Brodaty and Donkin 2009).

A real life profile of a person named anonymously as Aunt Mary is presented to give the reader a sense of the complexities of long-distance caregiving in an elderly relative who has developed the early symptoms of dementia.

9.3 What To Do About Aunt Mary?

It was early December, 2007 when my sister and I (JGB) wrote to our Aunt Mary about arranging our annual Christmas visit. We usually flew from Phoenix to Sacramento and rented a car to drive to Stockton where Aunt Mary had lived for over 50 years. She lived in the same house she had purchased new when she taught school in the Stockton area. Now retired for almost 30 years, she looked and acted much younger than her 98 years. She was the family's gatherer of news, pictures and made a point in keeping everyone connected. Her hand-written letters, often with newspaper clippings of stories or philosophy, could be counted on as regular as the church newsletter. We had made Christmas a time to spend with Aunt Mary as she lived alone and as the years left their limitations on her she found it difficult to travel to see her younger sisters and nieces and nephews and their children. So, family visited Aunt Mary often, but not often enough in our opinion. Holidays were special for our family, and we chose to accept Aunt Mary's invitation to visit. And we enjoyed our visits as Aunt Mary was a card player, puzzle solver, a witty storyteller, who enjoyed eating out, seeing the decorated homes at Christmas, and a fan of music and theater. We left our visits with Aunt Mary with sadness about their shortness; we felt uplifted and energized and grew in our love and respect for her.

We were surprised, therefore, not to receive any response to our letter to her; she was always so conscientious! We wondered about her well-being so we called her. "Why, of course," she said, she welcomed us and we agreed to arrive a few days before December 24th and stay until New Years. Her voice sounded a bit weak, but after all she was 98 years old.

---

[2] There is no clear-cut consensus regarding what constitutes long-term caregiving. Some have used a temporal definition describing distance in terms of the time required to reach the care recipient. Others use a spatial definition such as the miles between the caregiver's and care recipient's residences. Still others use a combination of travel time and geographic distance. Also the term "long-distance" covers a range of possible assistance from complex responsibility for care, providing some financial support, arrangement for various levels of care, regular visits and phone calls, and oversight of medical care. The quantity and quality of interactions may vary depending on distance and availability of resources.

We arrived at Aunt Mary's house about mid-afternoon on a typical Northern California winter day. The morning paper was still on the doorstep, unusual because Aunt Mary worked all the available puzzles in the morning paper every day after breakfast. It took some time after the doorbell and knocks on the door before Aunt Mary came to the door with her walker. She looked frail and thin and gave us tentative hugs so as not to lose her balance. We spent the evening catching up on family news and after a small snack, Mary excused herself and retired to her bedroom. We were surprised; she was always a conversationalist.

We noticed a pile of mail at one end of the kitchen table, a refrigerator that needed restocking, and the guest beds unprepared for us as they were in previous visits. It was 10:00 a.m. the next day, after my sister and I had had breakfast, that we decided to knock on Aunt Mary's bedroom door. She had always prepared breakfast for all of us before or suggested a visit to a local restaurant. It took about an hour for Aunt Mary to get ready for the day. We asked her how she was getting to the grocery store and getting to her hair and doctor's appointments. She said that she had been driving her 1966 Chevy Malibu to run errands, play bridge with friends, and maintain her appointments. While we were there we used the rental car which I drove as Aunt Mary occupied the front seat to give directions and caution me about speed. I felt unsafe just thinking about how she managed to drive her car with her degree of frailty and general alertness. After two days at Aunt Mary's my sister and I took a long walk in the neighborhood to discuss "What do we do about Aunt Mary?"

One of our biggest concerns was Aunt Mary's safety. While she lived in a cul-de-sac with neighbors who monitored each other's activities, the larger neighborhood had deteriorated and the residents more temporary. We knew Aunt Mary was adamant about staying in her house as she had turned down previous suggestions we had made about moving to an apartment or to live with one of us in Phoenix. Indeed, her friends were all in Stockton and weekly bridge had become the centerpiece of their social network. We discussed options to present to Aunt Mary, which included assisted living or getting a roommate to live with her. We had done some homework and heard of a local healthcare group called the Visiting Angels, which provided a variety of services in one's home on a daily or weekly basis. This option seemed to be the best one we thought as it respected Aunt Mary's autonomy, and was affordable. At least it was a first step given the shortness of our visit and it being a major holiday season. We presented our concern about safety to Aunt Mary when she awakened from a nap of several hours. We called Visiting Angels and the owner came to Aunt Mary's house within the hour to meet Mary and discuss our needs and possible arrangements. We agreed that a nurse's aide would visit Aunt Mary three times a week, do minor house cleaning, laundry, prepare lunch, and be a friend for 4 h each visit. The plan was put in place the week after Christmas.

Visiting Angels would inform me by email of how Aunt Mary was doing and any problems. I, too, would call Aunt Mary to get her opinion about this arrangement. Initially the Visiting Angels had to work out some issues related to time, tasks, and authority, but overall things worked well. I planned on returning to Stockton at least once a month.

There were several other issues besides safety that had to be addressed before we returned to Phoenix. One was the pile of mail on the kitchen table. When I asked Aunt Mary about the mail she said, “I didn’t know what to do with it so I put it in a pile on the table.” Not surprisingly bills had not been paid for several months and had grown substantially with late fees, and with repeated threats to cut off service. We learned from the yardman that electric service had been cut off, and following her call to the yardman to inform him, he had paid the bill. Similar threats existed for water and phone services. The yardman had asked Aunt Mary about any relatives at the time and Aunt Mary said that she had none. I sorted the mail, paid the bills before we returned to Phoenix and I informed Aunt Mary that I would have her mail forwarded to me and I would make out the checks for her to sign and mail. The biggest problem was what to do to get her multiple magazine subscriptions cancelled. She had been an easy target for magazine vendors for years.

Another key issue we needed to address was the car—Aunt Mary’s key possession. She talked about her car as if it were her child. California had just renewed her license at age 98! The car was a 1966 vintage model, Chevrolet with less than 100,000 miles, with the original paint and pampered; oil was changed religiously every 5,000 miles and recorded in a journal she kept in the glove box. The car drew many offers from young men when Aunt Mary filled up with gas at her usual gas station. In Aunt Mary’s eyes the car and she were inseparable, and was worth at least $ 20,000! But, after seeing Aunt Mary’s dependence on a walker and her slow reaction time while driving, I feared for her life and those lives of others, especially children near school zones. Even though we discussed her responsibilities as a car owner, several times heatedly, she said that she was going to continue to drive. She was not going to ask others for rides! And, besides how would she get to contract bridge each week to see her fellow card players who were in a local nursing home if she couldn’t drive? This problem could not be resolved during our Christmas visit, but I knew it would sneak up and bite us again, which it did.

Still another major issue to be addressed before we left for Phoenix was Aunt Mary’s healthcare. Aunt Mary had been blessed with good health during her lifetime needing only doctor visits for allergy shots. But, she never talked about her health; she never complained about aches and pains. She was not into cooking or following a balanced diet. This was apparent to us in her loss of weight and strength. We stressed with Visiting Angels the importance of getting her to buy more fresh fruit and vegetables on visits to the grocery store. However, Aunt Mary’s attitudes and habits were not easily changed. She was seeing a doctor and on medications for osteoarthritis; the doctor also referred her for physical therapy and nutritional services. We left feeling good about Aunt Mary’s healthcare even though her follow through was less than we had hoped for.

It’s now 2008 and we are back in Phoenix. I kept in touch with the Visiting Angels and also Aunt Mary. In February we celebrated Aunt Mary’s 99th birthday. We talked about making it to 100. She said the neighbors were planning to have a party for her then. The arrangements with the Visiting Angels were working well except there were some changes in the nurse’s aides causing some schedule changes and Aunt Mary would not let the aides prepare her meals. Instead Aunt Mary and the aide went to Mary's favorite sandwich shop where she could get homemade ice cream for dessert. And yes, despite my continuing objections, Aunt Mary was driving her car.

About April I received a call from Visiting Angels saying that Aunt Mary was hospitalized for dizziness, weakness and dehydration. I flew to California and, as usual, rented a car for the drive to Stockton. I found her sitting up in her hospital bed holding forth with several nurses who were surprised to see me as Aunt Mary had told them she had no living family members. The doctor told me to watch for falls and gave me a prescription. I took Aunt Mary home. She had a follow-up visit with her usual doctor a week later. I took her to that appointment. The doctor told Aunt Mary and me that she should be in an assisted living facility; he was concerned about her poor nutrition and risk of falling. Aunt Mary smiled politely. She was opposed to moving to a facility. I did some research on available, affordable assisted living facilities in the area. Meanwhile Aunt Mary agreed to increasing the coverage by the Visiting Angels to 5 h a day 5 days a week. I returned to Phoenix.

In June I returned to visit Aunt Mary and convinced her to visit three assisted living facilities that were within her budget. She was on California's teacher's retirement plan, which was modest to say the least. Aunt Mary never voiced an opinion about the facilities and it didn't matter because I later discovered that her health insurance would not help pay for assisted living, only nursing home care. So we settled for as much care from Visiting Angels as she could afford. I continued to worry about falls and her well-being over weekends. She seemed to be accepting of more visits by the Visiting Angels as long as she could stay in her home.

I had been back in Phoenix for about a month when I received a call from Visiting Angels alerting me that, in their opinion, Aunt Mary needed assisted living as she was becoming more frail and stubborn about doing what she wanted to do without asking for help. For some reason she felt more comfortable calling the yardman for help than her neighbors or the Visiting Angels. This is precisely who she called when she returned from an appointment to find her house had been burglarized. The yardman called me and the police. I quickly arranged a trip to Stockton.

While her house was ransacked it was apparent the thieves knew what they wanted and cleaned out her jewelry in an adjacent bedroom and her checkbook from her desk in her bedroom. The thieves had a plan to carry out the robbery during a 2-h block of time when she would be at a doctor's appointment. They had gained entrance through the unlocked side door on the garage and lifted the door in the garage off of its hinges to enter the house. It looked like a plan that was developed knowing Aunt Mary's schedule as she was at home most of the time. Aunt Mary's reaction to the loss of her jewelry was almost one of disinterest, stating that most of it was inexpensive costume jewelry. I returned to Phoenix after talking with the police and insurance adjuster.

In August I received a call from the Visiting Angels to say that Aunt Mary was in a car accident, but unhurt. I called her at home. She minimized the accident not recalling how it happened. She was returning home when she said she heard a noise but kept on driving. When she pulled into her driveway she had two shredded tires on the right side of the car and some minor scratches. Her neighbor, who happened to work for a tire business, replaced the tires for her. And that was the end of her story. At my next visit a few weeks later I sat down with Aunt Mary eye-to-eye and asked for the car keys. She refused despite my examples of how she as a former school teacher was putting school children at the nearby school at risk, she refused to discuss giving up the car. I lost my cool and accused her of being uncooperative. She seemed surprised by my anger and tears. It was then that I realized that I was trying to be rational to someone who wasn't and I apologized. That night, before I was to return to Phoenix, I removed her car keys from her purse and informed the Visiting Angels to take her wherever she needed to go, which they did. I knew, however, that Aunt Mary did not stop driving. Her neighbor said she told him, "He (referring to me) doesn't know I have another key!" We never discussed the topic again, although it was always on my mind.

The morning of October 30, 2008 I received a call from the Visiting Angels that the nurse's aide found Aunt Mary in the bathtub, her body was warm, but there was no pulse. The EMTs attempted resuscitation unsuccessfully. Aunt Mary had died peacefully in her own home alone as she would have wanted, but disappointed that she didn't reach 100! I knew what to do about Aunt Mary. She and I had made arrangements for her at a funeral home and cemetery on one of my visits to Stockton. It was also where many of her friends were buried. She had the last say in where she wanted to be.

My later reflections on my care of Aunt Mary included the impact of her progressive dementia on her and on me, emotionally and physically. We were both emotionally drained and had neglected our physical health. First, for a person as fiercely independent who strived to be proactive and in control, the advent of dementia symptoms must have been devastating to Aunt Mary, but she kept her fears to herself. The first clue that something was wrong was losing control over her handwriting. Her checkbook reflected this change. And, it explains why she was overwhelmed by the mail, especially the bills which needed checks to be mailed. The first clue to me that something was wrong was the abrupt termination of her letters, always frequent and carefully written. I was in denial of the fact that Aunt Mary had dementia as I recalled her lucid times and always perceived her "in charge" of her life. Also, being recently retired I could envision myself in the same predicament. She was one of my favorite aunts as we had a lot of academic, social, and community interests in common. Rarely did she complain about anything—she always looked the same to me.

Aunt Mary should have been in an assisted living facility, but she was so opposed to the idea of leaving and selling her home that doing that against her will would have been cowardly and certain to be a cause of her death. Had she survived I was going to ask her doctor about at home hospice care. It would have meant that Aunt Mary would have had to accept the fact that she might not live to be 100. But, the Visiting Angels organization served both Aunt Mary and me, as a geographically remote caregiver, well. We were blessed that Aunt Mary did not experience a fall, a stroke, or a disabling car accident. She did, in fact, have a legion of Visiting Angels who provided preventive care to a stubborn, but loving, lady who appreciated them all.

9.4 Level of Burden Index

The geographical distance between the primary family caregiver and the care recipient has been one of the factors that have given rise to the need for contracted or outsourced care. Also, the aging process and the changing needs of chronic diseases as they evolve have also required that caregivers gradually give more time to the direct care of their ill and/or aging family member. Increasing time away from work is not always an option, even when there are increasing concerns about the care recipient's safety and ability to live without constant supervision. *The demands upon the primary caregiver have been called "the burden of care."* For example, a study of the demands on caregivers 1 year after stroke found that caregivers reported adverse effects on their emotional health, social activities, leisure time, and family relationships (Anderson et al. 1995). A national caregiver survey found that caregiving has greater effects on dementia caregivers than non-dementia caregivers. Dementia caregivers are more involved in caregiving in terms of hours per week as well as the number of ADL and IADL tasks (Ory et al. 1999). Furthermore, the study showed that dementia caregivers are affected more negatively by their caregiving responsibilities in terms of employment complications, caregiver strain, mental and physical health problems, time for leisure and other family members, and family conflict. One would expect based on the greater burden of caregiving on dementia caregivers, that they would be more inclined to utilize formal contracted services than those caring for someone without dementia.

The measure of Level of Burden is based on an index derived from the amount of time caregivers spend per week helping the care recipient and the number/type of activities performed for the recipient. This measure is important because in a national survey (National Alliance for Caregiving and AARP 1997) it was found that the greater the level of caregiver burden, or intensity, the stronger the impact of caregiving has on caregivers' perceived health (regardless of age, gender, education, or other factors). The amount of time caregivers say they spend giving care ranges from less than 1 h per week to more than 40 h per week. In addition, they provide a variety of types of support ranging from no activities of daily living (ADLs) to more than four ADLs and three to five instrumental activities of daily living (IADLs). In order to measure intensity, the Level of Burden Index classified caregivers into one of five levels.

Each successive level involves a higher degree of caregiver responsibility or demand. Level 1 caregivers perform no ADLs and donate relatively few hours a week of care. Level 5 caregivers reflect those with the heaviest burden. They help with at least two ADLs and provide more than 40 h per week of care. Table 9.1 shows the distribution of caregivers in this study by the Level of Burden Index.

Table 9.1 shows that as the level of the caregiving burden increases the greater the number of caregiving hours are required per week and the more ADLs and IADLs are performed by the caregiver.[3]

---

[3] An analysis of National Institutes of Health funding found the strongest predictor of funding was disability-adjusted life years. In 2005 conditions receiving the most funding based on disease

Table 9.1 Caregivers by Level of Burden Index. (Source: *Family Caregiving in the U.S.*, Findings from a National Survey, National Alliance for Caregiving and AARP, April 2004, p. 21)

	Level 1	Level 2	Level 3	Level 4	Level 5
Total	33 %	17	15	21	10
9 + h per week	2 %	59 %	50 %	100 %	100 %
Mean hrs per week	3.5	9.8	12.0	33.1	87.2
Mean no. of IADLs	3.1	4.0	4.3	5.2	5.9
Mean no. of ADLs	0	0.4	2.2	2.9	4.2

Base: 1,247 caregivers in the U.S.
ADLs activities of daily living such as bathing, dressing and self-feeding, *IADLs* instrumental activities of daily living such as housework, managing money and shopping for groceries

9.5 Caregiving Structures: Levels of Specialized Care

9.5.1 Contracts

Many people are willing to voluntarily care for a parent or loved one without any promise of compensation. Even so, a growing number of people are entering into caregiver contracts (also called personal service or personal care agreements) with their family members.[4] Having such a contract has many benefits. It rewards the family member for doing the work. It can help alleviate tension between family members by making sure the work is fairly compensated. If the care recipient does not have enough money to pay his/her caregiver, there may be other sources of payment. For example, a long-term care insurance policy may cover family caregivers or there may be state or federal government programs that compensate family caregivers. For example, the Veterans Administration has a caregiver support line for questions or assistance with their services, which include adult healthcare centers, home-based primary care, skilled home care, homemaker and home health aid, respite care, and hospice care (U.S. Dept. of Veterans Affairs 2012).[5]

A caregiver contract is a legal contract that defines the rights and obligations with respect to the care recipient. Contracts are used to make the specifics of the caregiver-care recipient relationship clear. The contract may also define tasks which the caregiver is not expected to complete. For example, many home health service providers do not provide cleaning services.

It is estimated that more than 80 % of people in the workforce age 50 and over will need to arrange for the care of a parent or parents. Some will address this by

burden were AIDS, diabetes mellitus, and perinatal conditions. Depression, injuries and chronic obstructive pulmonary disease were the most underfunded. See Gillum et al. (2011).

[4] There is some evidence that different structures of caregiving exist in different cultures. For example, one study has found that African-American families with dependent elders use multiple caregivers and that families organize themselves through defined caregiving structures when providing care. For example, elderly dependent family members are often cared for by two or more people whose roles and responsibilities address their needs. See Dilworth-Anderson et al. (1999).

[5] See VA Caregiver Support at http://www.caregiver.va.gov/support_services.asp.

handling caregiving tasks themselves, even quitting their jobs to do so. Others will continue to work and be caregivers with the assistance of relatives or outsourced contract caregivers or assisted living facilities. This is particularly true when the care recipient lives in another city or state and can't or won't relocate.

9.5.2 Levels of Specialized Care

Some diseases complete their lifecycles quickly while other take years to fully evolve. For example, Alzheimer's disease can last as long as 20 years (Alzheimer's Association 2010). This may mean that family caregivers may need to seek out professional full-time caregivers and facilities that have the resources to provide more specialized levels of care as the care recipient's condition warrants. Also, since care recipients, especially the elderly, may have more than one ailment requiring attention it makes the search for a facility with caregivers who are trained to address multiple needs more difficult.

A national survey of 1,677 family caregivers showed that half of these caregivers performed medical/nursing tasks for care recipients with multiple chronic physical and cognitive conditions (Reinhard et al. 2012). Three out of four (78 %) of family caregivers were managing medications, and administering intravenous fluids and injections. Most (51 %) of these family caregivers believed that they were helping their family member avoid institutionalization. Indeed, the more tasks family caregivers performed, the more likely they were to report that those efforts allowed the care recipient to avoid nursing home placement. Depending on the illness history of the care recipient, their age, and their cognitive and physical levels of functioning, it may only be a matter of time before a tipping point is reached and some type of specialized caregiving will be needed for the majority of elders.

Table 9.2 lists various types of caregiving arrangements that are available beginning with in-home care, out-of-home care, residential care facilities and hospice care. These choices form a continuum ranging from the minimum amount of care needed to special care units for the total care of Alzheimer and other persons with dementia. Hospice services are available at all levels of care. Caregivers can obtain various types of services as the condition and abilities of their loved one dictates.

9.6 Emotional and Financial Costs of Long-term Care for Caregivers

One of the key findings from caregiving studies over the past several decades has been that family caregiving can have negative effects on the caregiver's own financial situation, retirement security, physical and emotional health, social networks and careers. This is particularly severe for caregivers of individuals who have complex, chronic health conditions and both functional and cognitive impairments (Zarit et al. 1985; Feinberg et al. 2011).

Table 9.2 Levels of Specialized Care. (Sources: http://www.helpguide.org/elder/respite_care.htm and http://www.alz.org/care/alzheimers-dementia-residential-facilities.asp)

In-Home Care
In-home services can be provided by volunteer or paid help, occasionally or on a regular basis. Services may last from a few hours to overnight, and may be arranged directly or through an agency. This choice enables the patient to remain in his or her own home, and can be invaluable for caregivers
Stimulation, recreation, and companionship can be provided by family members, friends, or neighbors while you take a break. Faith-based, community, and other non-profit organizations recruit volunteers, while home-care businesses provide trained staff to cover short in-home intervals
Personal care providers assist with daily living skills such as bathing, dressing, feeding, or toileting. *Homemaker services* support meal preparation, shopping, and housekeeping. *Skilled healthcare*, which requires more specialized training and experience, addresses medical needs
Out-of-Home Care
Adult day centers are for older adults who can no longer manage independently, or who are isolated and lonely. Planned activities promote well-being through social and health services. Adult day care centers operate during daytime hours, Monday through Friday, in a safe, supportive, and positive environment. Nutritious meals and snacks that accommodate special diets are typically included
Residential Care
Retirement housing may be appropriate for individuals who are able to care for themselves independently. A person may be able to live alone safely, but has difficulty managing an entire house. Generally, this type of senior housing provides limited supervision and may offer opportunities for social activities, transportation and other amenities
Continuing care retirement communities (CCRC)
CCRCs provide different levels of care (independent, assisted living and nursing home) based on individual needs. A resident is able to move throughout the different levels of care within the community if his or her needs change. Payment for these types of facilities can include an initial entry fee with subsequent monthly fees or payment may be based solely on monthly fees
Assisted living (also called residential care home, adult living, supported care)
Assisted living bridges the gap between living independently and living in a nursing home. Typically offers a combination of housing, meals, supportive services and healthcare. Assisted living residences generally provide 24-h staff, recreational activities, housekeeping, laundry and transportation. Residents may choose which services they receive from the facility such as help with bathing, dressing, eating or medication reminders. Costs depend on the services provided. The federal government does not regulate assisted living and definitions of assisted living vary from state to state. Assisted living facilities may or may not offer services designed for people with dementia
Nursing homes (also called skilled nursing facility, long-term care facility, custodial care)
Nursing homes provide 24 h care and long-term medical treatment. Most nursing homes have services and staff to address issues such as nutrition, care planning, recreation, spirituality and medical care. Different nursing homes have different staff-to-resident ratios. Also, the staff at one nursing home may have more experience or training than the staff at another. Nursing homes are usually licensed by the state and regulated by the federal government

Table 9.2 (continued)

Alzheimer special care units (SCUs) (also called memory care units)
SCUs meet the specific needs of individuals with Alzheimer's disease and other dementias. SCUs can take many forms and exist within various types of residential care. Such units most often are cluster settings in which persons with dementia are grouped together on a floor or a unit within a larger residential care facility. Some states have legislation requiring nursing homes and assisted living residences to tell exactly what specialized services their SCU provides, including a trained staff, specialized activities, and ability of staff to care for residents with behavioral needs
Hospice Care (services available at all levels of specialized care)
Directed at quality of life, hospice provides support for end-of-life care in the home or hospital (nursing care, physician care, medication management, psychosocial care, caregiver support and spiritual care). For-profit and not-for-profit hospices provide similar services

9.6.1 Financial Costs

Studies have found that from 24–60 % of caregivers report a moderate to high financial hardship as a result of caregiving. Many caregivers make direct out-of-pocket expenditures of 10 % or more of their annual income on caregiving expenses. Some caregivers are forced to leave the labor force and lose their benefits. There are economic consequences for employers in lost productivity and higher healthcare costs.

The vast majority of older adults with disabilities living in the community receive family care. However, in the most recent decade more families have been left to carry the burden alone as caregivers are not able to afford paid help in the home. As the care recipient's disability becomes more severe and more physically demanding, caregiver stress increases (Caswell 2004). Caregiver stress is a strong predictor of nursing home entry. There is strong interest in helping to delay or prevent nursing home use or unnecessary hospitalizations by improving family caregiving experiences. For caregivers of dementia patients there is growing consensus that more comprehensive and multicomponent interventions are needed. Recent interventions for caregivers of cancer patients have found significant, positive effects on multiple outcomes (Feinberg et al. 2011). There is interest in shifting away from institutional care to more home-based care if family support services were more available. (Conner 2007; Conner et al. 2007; Knee, 2010; Phillips et al. 2008).

9.6.2 Emotional Costs

While institutionalization might seem to be a "relief" or partial respite from the stress of home care, it has been found that caregivers who institutionalized a relative with dementia had depression and anxiety levels as high as they were while they were in-home caregivers (Schulz et al. 2004). The transition to institutionalized care was particularly difficult for spouses, almost half of whom visited their spouse daily and continued to provide help with physical care during their visits. One eventual outcome of a dementing illness on the marital relationship is that the relationship loses the potential for reciprocity and shared meaning. Women are more distressed in inequitable exchanges than men (Hooker et al. 2000). Caregivers of persons with moderate to severe dementia have higher burden indices, especially in the loss of control. This is not surprising since many behavior disturbances are more common as dementia progresses (Messinger-Rapport et al. 2006).

There is evidence that the consequences of long-term caregiving may be long-term as well. A 4-year longitudinal study of caregivers who had cared for a relative with progressive dementia found that caregivers continued to show higher rates of depression and anxiety disorders for as long as 3 years after bereavement (Bodnar and Kiecolt-Glaser 1994). Although greater loneliness may be a natural consequence of losing one's partner, the failure of former caregivers to return to baseline scores on anxiety and depression suggests that adjustment following a long period of caregiving may pose unique challenges (Robinson-Whelen et al. 2001). Indeed, where a person dies is part of the enduring memory a family will have of that person. A higher rate of concerns with the quality of end-of-life care has been reported for persons whose last place of care was a nursing home or hospital (Teno et al. 2004). Increasingly nursing homes are replacing hospitals as the last place of care. Bereaved family members have voiced concerns with the quality of end-of-life care regardless of where it was provided. Only bereaved family members whose loved one received home hospice services reported higher satisfaction and fewer unmet needs (Teno et al. 2004).

9.7 Summary

Family caregiving is now viewed as an important public health concern. Families remain the most important source of support and care to older adults. However, greater longevity with more complex chronic diseases has made family caregiving more physically and emotionally demanding. Family caregivers have little or no training to perform the tasks of caregiving. The financial costs and out-of-pocket expenses make it impossible to keep family members at home. Caregiving has become a full-time job for many.

Geographic and job mobility has made it necessary to engage in long distance caregiving, especially since it is often not possible for the care recipient to relocate. Nearly 69 % of caregivers have made accommodations at work because of caregiving. These adjustments have often affected income and made it necessary to reduce paid help. Some caregivers have left full-time employment. In addition, the stresses of caregiving have increased, in some cases caregivers have institutionalized family members, especially those with severe cognitive impairments.

The work of caregiving has a substantial impact on the health and well-being of caregivers. Between 40 and 70 % of caregivers develop clinical depression. Caregivers have poorer physical health than non-caregivers, and have more frequent visits to the emergency room or hospitalization. Nonetheless, families are key in managing the continuity of care for their loved ones.

It has become necessary to outsource care, especially specialized care as care recipients' needs change and they require 24 h care and supervision. The economic downturn and budget cuts have resulted in less family flexibility where they are able to financially place their relative. Trends suggest future reliance on fewer family caregivers. Disability levels of older adults living in the community continue to increase as does the age of family caregivers. Yet, there is a shift away from institutionalized care to home care. There is a great need for federal policy governing the supportive care of older, disabled, and impaired citizens.

9.8 Questions for Discussion

1. Are you now, or have you been, a long distance caregiver? What were the satisfactions and frustrations you experienced?
2. Describe the personal effects of learning that a family member has dementia, Parkinson's disease or other progressive, chronic disease.
3. What are some other approaches that could be used in the care of "Aunt Mary," the case illustration presented in the text?
4. Explain the Level of Burden Index.
5. What is meant by the continuum of care?

References

Alzheimer's Association. (2010). 2010 Alzheimer's disease facts and figures. http://www.alz.org/documents_custom/report_alzfactsfigures2010.pdf. Accessed 15 April 2014.

Anderson, C. S., Linto, J., & Stewart-Wynne, E. G. (1995). A population-based assessment of the impact and burden of caregiving for long-term stroke survivors. *Stroke; A Journal Of Cerebral Circulation, 26*(5), 843–849.

Bledsoe, L. K., Moore, S. E., & Collins, W. L. (2010). Long-distance caregiving: An evaluative review of the literature. *Ageing International, 35*(4), 293–310.

Bodnar, J. C., & Kiecolt-Glaser, J. K. (1994). Caregiver depression after bereavement: Chronic stress isn't over when it's over. *Psychology & Aging, 9*(3), 372–380.

Bookman, A., & Kimbrel, D. (2011). Families and elder care in the twenty-first century. *Work & Family, 21*(2), 117–140.

Brodaty, H., & Donkin, M. (2009). Family caregivers of people with dementia. *Dialogues in Clinical Neuroscience, 11*(2), 217–228.

Caswell, J. (2004). The job no one asks for. *Heartbeat, Summer,* 10–14.

Conner, S. R. (1997). *Hospice: Practice, pitfalls and promise*. Washington, DC: Taylor & Francis.

Conner, S. R., Pyenson, B., Fitch, K., Spence, C., & Iwasaki, K. (2007). Comparing hospice and nonhospice patient survival among patients who die within a three-year window. *Journal of Pain Symptom Management, 33,* 238–246.

Dilworth-Anderson, P., Williams, S. W., & Cooper, T. (1999). Family caregiving to elderly African Americas: Caregiver types and structures. *Journal of Gerontology, 54B*(4), 5237–5241.

Feinberg, L., Reinhard, S. C., Houser, A., & Choula, R. (2011). *Valuing the invaluable: 2011 Update contributions and costs of family caregiving*. Washington, DC: AARP Public Policy Institute.

Gillum, L. A., Gouveia, C., Dorsey, E. R., Pletcher, M., et al. (2011). NIH disease funding levels and burden of disease. *PLoS ONE, 6*(2), e16837. doi:10.1371/journal.pone.0016837.

Hochschild, A. R. (2012). *The outsourced self: Intimate life in market times*. New York: Metropolitan Books/Henry Holt & Co.

Hooker, K., Manoogian-O'Dell, M., Monahan, D. J., Frazier, L. D., & Shifren, K. (2000). Does type of disease matter? Gender differences among Alzheimer's and Parkinson's disease spouse caregivers. *The Gerontologist, 40*(5), 568–573.

Knee, D. O. (2010). Hospice care for the aging population in the United States. In J. C. Cavanaugh & C. K. Cavanaugh (Eds.), *Aging in America, Societal Issues* (Vol. 3, pp. 203–221). Denver: Praeger.

Koerin, B. B., & Harrigan, M. P. (2003). P.S. I love you! Long-distance caregiving. *Journal of Gerontological Social Work, 40*(1/2), 63–81.

Messinger-Rapport, B. J., McCallum, T. J., & Hujer, M. E. (2006). Impact of dementia caregiving on the caregiver in the continuum of care. *Long-Term Care: Clinical Care & Aging, 14*(1), 32–50.

Metlife Mature Market Institute and National Alliance for Caregiving. (2004). Miles away: The Metlife study of long-distance caregiving, July 2004. http://www.maturemarketinstitute.com. Accessed 9 October 2012.

Moore, M. J., Zhu, C. W., & Clipp, E. C. (2001). Informal costs of dementia care. Estimates from the National Longitudinal Caregiver Study. *Journal of Gerontology Series B: Psychological Sciences and Social Sciences, 56*(4), S219–S228.

National Alliance for Caregiving and AARP. (1997). Family caregiving in the U.S. National Alliance for Caregiving and AARP. Final Report, June 1997. http://assets.aarp.org/rgcenter//il/caregiving_97.pdf. Accessed January 2012.

Neal, M. B., Wagner, D. L., Bonn, K. J. B., & Niles-Yokum, K. (2008). Caring from a distance: Contemporary care issues. In A. Martin-Matthews & J. E. Philips (Eds.), *Aging and caring at the intersection of work and home life: Blurring the boundaries* (pp. 107–128). New York: Lawrence Erlbaum.

Ory, M. G., Hoffman, R. R., Yee, J. L., Tennstedt, S., & Schulz, R. (1999). Prevalence and impact of caregiving: A detailed comparison between dementia and nondementia caregivers. *The Gerontologist, 39*(2), 177–185.

Philips, J. E., & Martin-Matthews, A. (2008). Blurring the boundaries: Aging and caring at the intersection of work and home life. In A. Martin-Matthews & J. E. Philips (Eds.), *Aging and caring at the intersection of work and home life: Blurring the boundaries* (pp. 245–254). New York: Laurence Erlbaum.

Reinhard, S. C., Levine, C., & Samis, S. (2012). Home alone: Family caregivers providing complex chronic care. Funded by AARP Public Policy Institute and United Hospital Fund, October 2012. AARP Public Policy Institute, Washington, DC. http://www.aarp.org/ppi.

Robinson-Whelen, S., Tada, Y., MacCallum, R. C., McGuire, L., & Kiecolt-Glaser, J. (2001). Long-term caregiving: What happens when it ends? *Journal of Abnormal Psychology, 110*(4), 573–584.

Schultz, R., Belle, S. H., Czaia, S. J., Stevens, A., & Zhang, S. (2004). Long-term care placement of dementia patients and caregiver health and well-being. *Journal of the American Medical Association, 292*(8), 961–967.

Teno, J. M., Clarridge, B. R., Casey, V., Welch, L. C., Wetle, T., Shield, R., & Mor, V. (2004). Family perspectives on end-of-life care at the last place of care. *Journal of the American Medical Association, 291*(1), 88–93.

U.S. Department of Veterans Affairs Caregiver Support. http://www.google.com/search?client=safari&ris+en&g=U.S.+Department of Veterans+Affairs+Caregiving&le=UTF. Accessed 27 April 2014.

Zarit, S. H., Orr, N. K., & Zarit, J. M. (1985). *The hidden victims of Alzheimer's disease: Families under stress*. New York: New York University Press.

Chapter 10
Caregiving at the End of Life

10.1 Introduction

"Dying is hard. Most people die in a hospital. This, in itself is the primary reason that dying is so hard… The hospital is not by definition set up to meet the needs of people whose physical condition is beyond the capability for successful intervention…There is nothing in the system that provides for human nurturance to the soul when the body is beyond repair" (Kübler-Ross 1973, p. 6).

The place of death is one indicator of the kind of end-of-life care a dying person will experience (Flory et al. 2004). Not too long ago people used to die at home among family members. By the 1980s most dying moved out of the home into medical institutions (Kaufman 2005; McLeod 1999). How we die is another indicator of end-of-life care (Nuland 1993).[1] People used to die more naturally without being connected to multiple artificial life-sustaining measures. In medical institutions there is a culture of trying to stave off death with technological interventions. With the process of dying often prolonged and increasingly institutionalized there are serious concerns on behalf of dying patients about costs and experiencing a good death (National Institute on Aging 2008).

The majority of Americans die in a hospital or nursing home (Byock 2012). Total healthcare costs in the U.S. exceeded $ 2.6 trillion in 2010 and are expected to continue to rise in the foreseeable future with a disproportional share spent at the end of life.[2] In 2008, 28 % or $ 101 billion of total Medicare spending occurred during the last 2 months of life (USA Inc. 2011).

A good death was once a matter of luck, simply because some terminal illnesses were more painful and debasing than others (Webb 1997). Today, people want death to be made comfortable by the tools of medicine (Kaufman 2005). However, a good death has more to do with the decisions we make about our medical treatment and terminal care. What people fear most is a painful, protracted death, and dying alone.

---

[1] Also see, Buchwald (2006). Also, Albom (1997).

[2] See *President's Commission for the Study of Ethical Problems in Medicine and Biomedical and Behavioral Research* (1978–1983). Library of Congress card number 81-600150. Superintendent of Documents, U.S. Government Printing Office, Washington DC.

J. G. Bruhn, H. M. Rebach, *The Sociology of Caregiving*,
Clinical Sociology: Research and Practice, DOI 10.1007/978-94-017-8857-1_10,

Today, death is often complicated. Patients can choose or change the focus of their care from treatment to comfort and elect to receive palliative or hospice services in a growing number of healthcare settings. Many people want to control the way death happens for themselves and their loved ones by planning ahead, yet few are prepared for the time when decisions must be made (Kaufman 2005).

Communication between patients, families and providers is important across the span of end-of-life-care (Hooyman and Kramer 2006). A recent study showed that end-of-life conversations between patients and physicians were associated with fewer life-sustaining procedures and lower rates of intensive care unit admissions. Patients with advanced cancer who reported having end-of-life conversations with their physicians had significantly lower healthcare costs in their final week of life. Higher care costs near the end of life rise exponentially. Patients with higher costs had a worse quality of death in their final week (Zhang et al. 2009). This study pointed out the importance of palliative care both in reducing healthcare costs for the terminally ill and facilitating an environment conducive to experiencing a good death.[3] Two physicians who practice palliative care have stated, "What is certain is that palliative care must be integrated into the overall care of all end-stage organ diseases, if we want our patients and families to receive the best care possible throughout the spectrum of their illnesses." (Liao and Arnold 2007, p. 184).

Hospitals are not structured for the kinds of deaths that people claim to want. For example, Medicare's reimbursement methods dominate what happens to the majority of hospital patients at the end of life. In an attempt to control spending Medicare has been eliminating its cost-based payments to hospitals and nursing homes, and hospitals are not explicitly reimbursed for providing palliative care. The institutional response to these cutbacks has been for nursing homes to transfer dying patients to hospitals to avoid the cost of intensive treatment, and for hospitals to discharge patients, once they are labeled "dying" so as not to incur the cost of palliative care (Kaufman 2005, p. 29).

Palliative and hospice care are alternative pathways that do not prolong death for the patient but acknowledge death's inevitability. Dying today is about making choices early in a patient's illness journey. Hospital death will continue to be problematic because hospital culture is historically based on overcoming disease and even old age itself. We need to provide choices in the process of dying that address individual's needs and respect their autonomy (Kaufman 2005, pp. 320–321).

[3] According to McWebb (1997) an environment for a good death has the following ten things in common: (1) open, ongoing conversation; (2) preservation of the patient's decision-making power; (3) sophisticated symptom control; (4) limits are set on excessive treatment; (5) a focus on preserving patient quality of life; (6) emotional support; (7) financial support; (8) family support; (9) spiritual support; and (10) the patient is not abandoned by the medical staff even when curative treatment is no longer required.

10.2 Definitions

10.2.1 Palliative Care and Hospice Care

Palliative care is specialized medical care for people with serious illnesses. It is focused on providing patients with relief from the symptoms, pain, and the stress of a serious illness whatever the prognosis. The goal is to improve the quality of life for both the patient and the family. Palliative care is appropriate for patients in all diverse stages, including those undergoing treatment for curable diseases and those living with chronic diseases, as well as patients who are nearing the end of life. Palliative care utilizes a multidisciplinary approach and team in formulating a plan of care to relieve patients' suffering.

Hospice is considered to be the model for quality, compassionate care for people facing a life-limiting illness or injury. It involves a team approach to medical care, pain management, and emotional and spiritual support tailored to meet patient's needs and wishes. Support is available to the family as well. The core of hospice and palliative care is the belief that each person has the right to die pain free and with dignity, and that families will receive the necessary support to allow us to do so. Typically a family member serves as the providing caregiver and helps make decisions for the terminally ill individual (National Hospice and Palliative Care Organization 2010).[4] Hospice staff is on-call 24 h a day, 7 days a week.

Figure 10.1 shows the distribution of Medicare certified hospice providers by state in 2010. There are about 5,000 hospice programs today located in all 50 states. The majority are independent, freestanding agencies. The remaining agencies are either part of a hospital system, home health agency, or nursing home. The primary diagnoses are shown in Table 10.1.

When hospice care in the United States was established in the 1970s, cancer patients made up the largest percentage of hospice admissions. Today, cancer diagnoses account for less than half of all hospice admissions (40.1 %). Currently, less than 25 % of U.S. deaths are now caused by cancer, with the majority of deaths due to other terminal diseases. The top four non-cancer primary diagnoses for patients admitted to hospice in 2009 were debility unspecified (13.1 %), heart disease (11.5 %), dementia (11.2 %), and lung disease (8.2 %).

10.2.2 End-of-Life and End-of-Life-Care

End-of-life is considered to be the period of time marked by disability or disease that is progressively worse until death. It is considered to be the final stage of the journey of life.

[4] See the excellent, helpful *Caregiver Handbook, The Four Stages of Caregiving* (Stage 1 Getting Started; Stage 2 Finding Help; Stage 3 Heavy Care and Stage 4 Letting Go) available to download and print from Area Agency on Aging of Paseo-Pinellas, Inc. at http://www.agingcarefl.org/caregiver/fourStages/toc.

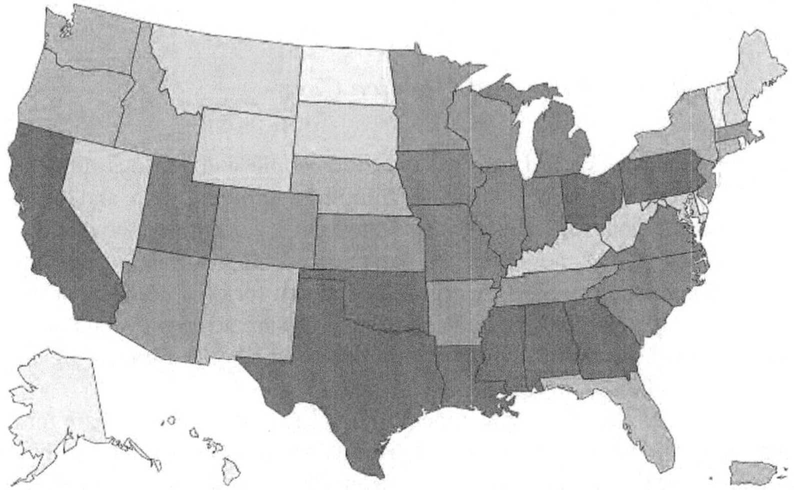

Fig. 10.1 Medicare certified hospices by state. (Source: National hospice and palliative care organization, NHPCO figure, 2010 edition, p. 10)

Table 10.1 Percentage of hospice admissions by primary diagnosis in 2009. (Source: NHPCO Facts and figures: *Hospice Care in America*, 2010 edition, p. 8)

Primary diagnosis	2009
Cancer	40.1 %
Non-cancer diagnoses	59.9 %
Debility unspecified	13.1 %
Heart disease	11.5 %
Dementia	11.2 %
Lung disease	8.2 %
Other	4.5 %
Stroke or coma	4.0 %
Kidney disease (ESRD)	3.8 %
Non-ALS motor neuron	1.9 %
Liver disease	1.8 %
HIV/AIDS	0.4 %
Amyotrophic lateral sclerosis (ALS)	0.4 %

End-of-life care is the care provided to a person in their final stages of life. It is also known as hospice care, comfort care, supportive care, palliative care, or symptom management (National Institutes of Health, 2006).

10.3 Where We Die

It is noteworthy that, while most Americans prefer to die at home, 60–70% still die in hospitals (Flory et al. 2004; Weitzen et al. 2003). Despite the existence of hospice as a Medicare benefit for over three decades, and numerous judicial rulings that have expanded patients' rights to terminate life-sustaining interventions, the program remains underused (Flory et al. 2004). Even though hospice care has grown dramatically, about 1 million people die each year without ever having access to hospice services (Morrison et al. 2008). Only 25% of Americans who died in 2000 were under hospice care at the time of death (Han et al. 2006). Even among Medicare decedents with end stage cancer diagnoses, only 44% used hospice care in 1996 (Virnig et al. 2002). And for those who used hospice in 2009 the median length of stay was only 21 days (NHPCO 2010). Hospice and palliative care programs can save hospitals between $ 1,700 and 4,900 per admission, ensure that patients receive individual, compassionate care, and increase patient satisfaction with their care (Brumley et al. 2007).

Hospice and palliative care may prolong the lives of some terminally ill patients. In a 2010 study lung cancer patients receiving early palliative care lived 23.3% longer than those who delayed palliative care. Median survival for earlier palliative care patients was 2.7 months longer than those receiving standard care. The study authors stated that with earlier referral to a hospice program, patients may receive care that results in better management of symptoms, leading to a stabilization of their condition and prolonged survival (Ternel et al. 2010).

Several surveys of physicians' attitudes toward the use of hospice have found that male physicians have less favorable attitudes toward hospice than female physicians. Oncologists have less favorable attitudes than internists. Physicians without board certification also report less positive attitudes toward hospice care than board certified physicians (Bradley et al. 2002). The authors suggest targeted educational interventions among certain specialists may help change reluctant physicians. A more recent national survey of physicians and consumers found that the timing of end-of-life discussions between patients and physicians was key to the use of hospice services. There are key differences between physicians and patients when it comes to initiating the conversation. Physicians frequently wait until all treatment options have been exhausted to even bring up the topic. Patients would like to begin the conversation at the time of diagnosis or start of treatment (Crossroads Hospice 2011). These studies emphasize the importance of beginning the physician-patient-family end-of-life conversation at the time of diagnosis so that the decisions made become part of the total care plan. The patient and his/her primary caregiver have opinions, questions, are searching for support and reassurance, and need to be included in the visit when the physician's diagnosis/prognosis is presented.

Nuland (1993), a surgeon, pointed out that the personality of the physician, particularly the need to control, is a factor in the dying process. "A doctor may maintain a bit of authority by exerting his authority over the dying process, which he does by controlling the duration and determining the moment at which he allows it to end. In this way, he deprives the patient and family of the control that is rightfully theirs. These days, many hospitalized patients die only when a doctor has decided that the right time has come" (p. 259).

10.4 The Trajectories of Dying

The concept of a trajectory of dying is often used to point out similarities and differences in patient experiences as they approach death (Field and Cassel 1997). The dying trajectory of each patient has at least two properties—duration and shape. Three possible trajectories toward death also help in understanding some of the common and different phases of caregiving at the end of life.[5]

Some people die suddenly and unexpectedly; others have forewarning. Those who die suddenly, for example, in an accident or of a heart attack, usually require primary caregiving bereavement for survivors. If a patient is admitted to a hospital emergency room at the time of death, there is usually a social worker present who calls the hospital chaplain and, together, they assist the family with grief support and planning.

Among those with a forewarning of death some steadily and predictably decline and at each stage of decline need additional care and close monitoring. This may require the transfer from home to a medical facility or hospice, or the transfer from a medical facility to a hospice or home, depending on resources, caregivers, and patient and family wishes. Other people may have long periods of chronic illness punctuated by crises, one of which may prove fatal, although an entirely new problem may intervene to cause death. These patients may understand that they have an incurable progressive illness that will likely kill them, but they may not see themselves—or be considered by their families—as dying (Field and Cassel 1997).

Those patients with forewarning of death may be differentiated from those who are imminently dying (likely to die in days) and those who are terminally ill, but not "actively" dying (not currently in the process of dying). These differences are important because they signal healthcare providers and family to attend to different clinical and personal priorities. Differences are also important because Medicare coverage for hospice services, which are specifically for dying patients, requires a medical determination that a patient has a terminal illness and has 6 months or less to live.

Depending on the nature of the illness and the patient's circumstances, the end of life may last a matter of days or months. During this time palliative care measures can provide the patient with pain control and other symptoms, such as constipation, nausea, or shortness of breath. Caregivers can find the last stages uniquely challenging. End-of-life caregiving requires support from a variety of sources.

There isn't a single specific point in an illness when end-of-life care begins; it depends on the individual. In the case of Alzheimer's disease, the patient's physician

[5] Also see Lynn (2005).

can provide a caregiver with information on stages in the diagnosis. These stages can provide general guidelines for understanding the progression of Alzheimer's symptoms and planning care. Yet, illness progression depends on many individual factors (Wayne et al. 2012).

When caregivers and family members are clear about a patient's preferences for treatment in the final stages of life, they can devote their time to comfort care. A terminally ill patient's deteriorating physical condition, increased physical safety needs, and the 24-h demands of final stage care often means that the primary caretaker will need additional in-home help or for the patient to be admitted to an inpatient hospice. In many cases, patients prefer to remain at home in comfortable and familiar surroundings with family. Hospice personnel can continue to provide assistance in the patient's home or onsite at some hospitals, nursing homes or other facilities. When hospice care is provided at home a hospice team provides emotional and spiritual support according to the wishes of the patient and family. They also offer emotional support to the patient's family including grief counseling (Bumagin and Hirn 2001).

While the symptoms in the final stages will vary from patient to patient and according to their illness, there are some common symptoms experienced near the end of life that caregivers can recognize and provide comfort for: drowsiness; becoming unresponsive; confusion about time, place, and identity of loved ones; loss of appetite and decreased need for food and fluids; loss of bladder or bowel control; skin becoming cool to the touch; and labored, irregular, shallow or noisy breathing (Wayne et al. 2012).

The end-of-life period, when death is imminent, usually lasts from a few days to a few weeks. Some patients give up more readily than others. Decisions about hydration, breathing support, and other interventions should be consistent with the patient's and family's wishes.

A longitudinal cohort of 396 advanced cancer patients were followed prospectively to their death to determine the most influential set of factors that predict the quality of life at the end of life (Zhang et al. 2012). Two of the most important determinants of *poor* patient quality of life at the end of life were hospitalizations and admission to intensive care. The predictors of the *best* quality of life at the end of life were: (1) patients who engaged in prayer or meditation and made use of pastoral care services; (2) patients who felt treated with respect and as "a whole person" by their physician; and (3) physicians who were able to remain engaged and "present" for their dying patients (therapeutic alliance).

10.5 Men as Caregivers

Men are playing greater roles as caregivers. Men constitute about one-third of family caregivers (Arber and Gilbert 1989). Husbands, in particular, are encountering role transformations as they witness their wives grow in dependence as a result of age and chronic health conditions. Despite their effectiveness as caregivers, studies of male caregivers have found that they are not immune to the strains of caregiving including depression, grief, and burden, and the need for assistance from support networks. Men learn at an early age to be self-sufficient; asking for assistance is considered a sign of weakness. Yet, research has shown that men possess a strong sense of duty to the care recipient using a problem-solving process (Sanders and Power 2009; Watson 2010; Kramer and Thompson 2002). The male caregiving style has been described as "a model of caregiving that blends management with nurturing" (Russell 2001, p. 360). Yet, it is misleading to attribute differences in caregiving approaches, styles, or outcomes to sex difference without consideration for contextual factors such as how caregivers cope with the demands of their roles and how gender operates as a mediating variable linking coping and burden (Baker and Robertson 2008). Furthermore, the majority of studies of men as caregivers have focused on how male caregivers cope with people with dementia or other cognitively impaired adults where reciprocity is minimal or nil. We need more information about men's reciprocity experiences within their family.

Reciprocity, or the exchange of resources, is a dimension of social support that is important in caregivers' ability to sustain supportive relationships while caregiving. Caregivers of cognitively impaired older adults can experience difficulty in maintaining reciprocity in their relationships with care recipients who are unable to communicate. In a focus group study of 22 male caregivers giving care to cognitively impaired persons, Neufeld and Harrison (1998) found that men who focused on unique aspects of the recipient as a person or who expressed a high commitment to altruistic values had more positive feelings about their caregiving experience. However, most of the men described their caregiving on the basis of obligation or responsibility without any form of reciprocity.

10.5.1 Men as Caregivers at the End-of-Life

Few studies have focused on men as caregivers at the end-of-life. Fromme et al. (2005) interviewed a sample of 1,384 caregivers from a pool of 3,048 Oregon death certificates to examine caregiver strain at the end-of-life. Men constituted 29 % of the sample. As caregiver at the end-of-life men were less common, less likely to report caregiver distress and decedent symptom distress. Analysis revealed that men used fewer words than women to describe their experiences and only 15 % of men mentioned their own struggles. As caregivers at the end-of-life, men were less common and less likely to report caregiver strain and decedent symptom distress. Healthcare professionals should actively ask men about these issues and listen carefully, as their responses may be brief and understated.

Martin and Doka (2000), in their book, *Men Don't Cry … Women Do*, describe how overly expressing emotion and consciously seeking support is only one pattern or way of experiencing grief in our society. They describe two patterns of grieving. One is *intuitive* or affective, a second way is *instrumental*—it is experienced physically. The instrumental pattern is the way many men grieve due to male socialization. Women may also exhibit an instrumental style. But, the authors point out, patterns are *influenced* by gender not *determined* by it (p. 2).

Martin and Doka state that there are many facets of loss which are experienced at many levels—physical, emotional, cognitive, and spiritual—and are expressed and observable in a variety of behavior. In many instances responses will be blended. Similarly, caregiving at the end-of-life will be experienced differently by different caregivers.

10.6 Impact of End-of-life Care on Caregivers

End-of-life care poses unique challenges in intensity, which are usually specific to the nature of the disease and to the patient's level of disability. In particular, there are special challenges in the care of patients with cognitive impairment with respect to communication, pain control, and the need for extraordinary vigilance. A study of end-of-life care for patients with dementia showed that care was extremely demanding of caregivers (Schulz et al. 2003). Half of the caregivers reported spending at least 46 h per week assisting patients with activities of daily living. More than half of the caregivers reported that they felt they were "on duty" 24 h a day and they had to end or reduce their employment owing to the demands of caregiving. Caregivers showed high levels of depression while providing care to their relative with dementia, but showed remarkable resilience after death. Within 3 months of the death, the caregivers had clinically significant declines in their level of depression, and within 1 year depressive symptoms were lower than the levels reported while they were caregiving. Seventy-two percent of caregivers reported that the death was a relief for them, and more than 90 % reported the belief that it was also a relief to the patient. Therefore, only a minority of caregivers reported needing bereavement services. In contrast, caregivers whose relatives were institutionalized did not show an early and gradual recovery from depression. The authors point out several recommendations following their study. First, the need for support after a death is limited to a minority of caregivers which suggests that bereavement resources could be targeted. Second, when death is preceded by a protracted and stressful period of caregiving, it may be useful to offer bereavement resources to caregivers and family prior to, as well as after, the death occurs. Research suggests that the caregiving experiences of family members influence their adjustment to the patient's eventual death (Rabow et al. 2004). Caregiving support may be even more important than grief support.

10.7 Preventing Caregiver Burnout

Caregiving can be lonely, frustrating, stressful, and taxing—emotionally, physically, and financially (Carter 1994). At first most caregivers accept their new role as a caregiver with a sense of idealism, hope, and eagerness to do well. As time passes and the patient deteriorates and the caregiving demands increase in duration and intensity, fatigue sets in along with disappointments and frustration. *Caregiving burnout or compassion fatigue is a sense of being completely overwhelmed and unrewarded and is a common feeling among caregivers*. Feeling "burned out" can be harmful. Feeling stressed over long periods will affect one's health, motivation, mood, and attitude as well as the ability to cope with your own daily responsibilities. Sometimes the signs of burnout may not appear until after a patient's death, but they should be part of a caregiver's awareness from the onset of caregiving.

Caregiver burnout is the result of:

- Having difficulty asking for help
- High expectations of yourself and others
- A strong, unrealistic dedication to making things ideal for the person you are caring for
- Difficulty in saying "no"
- Consistently sacrificing yourself and your needs for the benefit of others
- Feeling as though you are the only person capable of providing care (Strom 2000; American Heart Association 2012)

Common emotional symptoms of burnout are:

- Becoming easily irritated and frustrated
- Feeling anger or resentment
- Sadness and feelings of loneliness
- Feeling overwhelmed and overloaded
- Decreased self esteem
- Depression
- Feeling emotionally drained (Strom 2000; American Heart Association 2012)

There are actions caregivers can take to minimize burnout and exhaustion:

- Accept one's limitations. Accept help. It is ok to say "no"
- Schedule breaks and private time. Eat well, get sleep, and exercise
- Take advantage of respite care usually provided by hospice volunteers
- Join a caregiver's support group in person or via the web
- Appreciate your own efforts. Define your limits
- Keep connected spiritually
- Communicate with family members
- Reflect on positive memories with the patient
- After the patient's death reconnect with others, acquire new skills, stay physically active, use your knowledge and experience to help others, talk to a therapist or counselor. Take care of yourself.

10.8 After Death Care for Caregivers

The effects of caregiving can extend beyond the death and burial of a loved one and can turn into a full depression and continued grief. Data suggest that some consequences of long-term caregiving may be long-term as well. A longitudinal study focused on what happened to caregivers in the years after their cognitively impaired spouse died. It was found that over a 4 year period former caregivers did not improve on several measures of psychological well-being. Although former caregivers experienced decreases in stress and negative affect, their scores on depression, loneliness and positive affect did not rebound to levels comparable to non-caregivers and, in fact, remained similar to those of current caregivers up to 3 years after caregiving had ceased (Tada et al. 2001).

When caregiving consumes the caregiver's life it erodes their identity forcing the caregiver to reestablish their needs and identity. Grieving can be therapeutic in the healing of the loss of the quality of life lost while caring for a loved one. Days of special meaning involving the deceased such as birthdays or anniversaries may reawaken the memories of the deceased loved one. Known as "anniversary reactions," it is normal to experience sadness during these times even for several years. Anticipation of these times can help caregivers to focus on positive memories and not become overwhelmed by grief and remorse. It is important for family caregivers to reestablish boundaries, reconnect with their identity, and find their spirit and inner strength.

The process of grieving and healing from long term caregiving takes time. It is important to take the time one needs to work through sorrow. Hospice offers the assistance of bereavement counseling for a year following a death. Helpful activities in working through sorrow include journaling, writing prose or poetry, taking a vacation, exercising, community service, meditation, relaxation and laughter. Caregiving is something most of us will do more than once in our lives, so we need to become better in integrating it into our lives.

10.9 Summary

The majority of Americans die in a hospital where the culture is oriented around prolonging life and curing disease. Also, hospitals are costly. Yet, many people want to control the way death happens for themselves and their loved ones. Hospice is growing in its use among the public and among some physicians, but only 25 % of Americans who died in 2000 were under hospice care at the time of death. Some physicians prefer to wait until all treatment options have been tried before a hospice referral, while many patients would like to explore options for their terminally ill family member at the time the diagnosis is made. The average length of time patients remain in hospice is about 21 days, too short to experience the array of services available for their care.

Caregiving at the end of life can follow one of three trajectories of dying. Some patients die suddenly, others experience a steady but predictable decline, while still others have long periods of illness interspersed by crises, one of which proves fatal. The demands on family caregivers differ in duration and intensity. Caregivers' adaptability can be taxed to the degree that they may become ill and even die before the person whom they are caring for. Caregivers experience both positive and negative effects of caregiving.

There isn't a single point in an illness when caregiving begins, and while it ends at death for the care recipient, caregivers' recovery can extend for months or even years. Most family caregivers are not trained for what they do; this can make the tasks of caregiving more difficult. Most caregivers are women, but almost one-third of family caregivers are men. Men are effective caregivers yet they are not immune to the strains of caregiving. Most men describe their caregiving on the basis of responsibility and obligation without expectations of reciprocity. There have been few studies of men as caregivers, especially at the end of life. One study found that men who were caregivers at the end of life did not talk about their stress and did not readily seek assistance or support.

Preventing caregiver burnout is a high priority in caregiving. Caregiver burnout or compassion fatigue is a sense of being overwhelmed and unrewarded and is a common feeling among caregivers. Feeling stressed over long periods will affect one's health, motivation, mood, and attitude as well as the ability to function as a caregiver. Signs and symptoms of burnout are presented and actions to minimize burnout are offered.

The effects of the care recipient's death can continue past the caregiving duties. The greatest loss for the caregiver is often their identity. The process of grieving and healing from long term caregiving takes time. Suggestions about coping with loss after loss are discussed.

10.10 Questions for Discussion

1. What is meant by a "good death"? Discuss.
2. What are some of the methodological difficulties in answering the question "Is caregiving harmful to one's health"? Discuss.
3. What are some of the barriers to getting hospice more accepted in our society? Discuss.
4. Explain the connection between where one dies and how one dies? Discuss.
5. What is needed to get more men to become caregivers in our society? Discuss.
6. Discuss the reasons why you think more ethnic minorities don't use hospice services?

References

Albom, M. (1997). *Tuesdays with Morrie*. New York: Doubleday.

American Heart Association. (2012). Signs of caregiver burnout. http://www.heart.org/HEARTORG/Caregiver/Responsiblities/SignsofcaregiverBurnout/Signs-of-Caregiver-Burnout_UCM_301831_Article.jsp. Accessed 6 January 2012.

Arber, S., & Gilbert, N. (1989). Transitions in caring: Gender, life course and the care of the elderly. In B. Bytheway, T. Keil, P. Allout, & B. Bytheway (Eds.), *Becoming and being old* (pp. 72–92). London: Sage.

Baker, K. L., & Robertson, N. (2008). Coping with caring for someone with dementia: Reviewing the literature about men. *Aging & Mental Health, 12*(4), 413–422.

Bradley, E. H., Cramer, L. D., Bogardus, S. T., Kasl, S. V., Johnson-Hurzeler, R., & Horowitz, S. M. (2002). Physicians' ratings of their knowledge, attitudes and end-of-life care practices. *Academic Medicine, 77*(4), 305–311.

Brumley, R., Enguidanos, S., Jamison, P., Seitz, R., Morgenstern, N., Saito, S., McIlwane, J., Hillary, K., & Gonzalez, J. (2007). Increased satisfaction with care and lower costs: Results of a randomized trial of in-home palliative care. *Journal of the American Geriatric Society, 55*(7), 993–1000.

Buchwald, A. (2006). *Too soon to say goodbye*. New York: Random House.

Bumagin, V. E., & Hirn, K. F. (2001). *Caregiving: A guide for those who give care and those who receive it*. New York: Springer.

Byock, I. (2012). *The best care possible*. New York: Avery.

Carter, R. (1994). *Helping yourself help others: A book for caregivers*. New York: Times Books.

Crossroads hospice. (2011). Are physicians and consumers on the same page about hospice? http://hospicecareresearch.blogspot.com/2011/05/are-physicians-and-consumers-on-same.html. Accessed 1 February 2011.

Field, M. J., & Cassel, C. K. (Eds.). (1997). *Approaching death: Improving care at the end of life*. Washington, D.C.: National Academy Press.

Flory, J., Young-Xu, Y., Gurol, I., Levinsky, N., Ash, A., & Emanuel, E. (2004). Place of death: U.S. trends since 1980. *Health Affairs, 23*(3), 194–200.

Fromme, E. K., Drach, L. L., Tolle, S. W., Ebert, P., Miller, P., Perrin, N., & Tilden, V. P. (2005). Men as caregivers at the end of life. *Journal of Palliative Medicine, 8*(6), 1167–1175.

Han, B., Remsburg, R. E., McAuley, W. J., Keay, T. J., & Travis, S. S. (2006). National trends in adult hospice use: 1991–1992 to 1999–2000. *Health Affairs, 25*(3), 792–799.

Hooyman, N. R., & Kramer, B. J. (2006). *Living through loss: Interventions across the life span*. New York: Columbia University Press.

Kaufman, S. R. (2005). *…And a time to die: How American hospitals shape the end of life*. Chicago: University of Chicago Press.

Kramer, B. J., & Thompson, E. H. (Eds.). (2002). *Men as caregivers*. New York: Prometheus Books.

Kübler-Ross, E. (1973). *Death: The final stage of growth*. Englewood Cliffs: Prentice-Hall.

Liao, S., & Arnold, R. M. (2007). Heart failure and the future of palliative medicine. *Journal of Palliative Medicine, 10*(1), 184.

Lynn J. (2005). Living long in fragile health: The new demographics shape end-of-life care. *Improving end of life care: Why has it been so difficult?* Hastings Center Report Special Report 35, no. 6 (2005) S14–S18.

Martin, T. L., & Doka, K. J. (2000). *Men don't cry…women do*. Philadelphia: Brunner/Mazel.

McLeod, B. W. (1999). *Caregiving: The spiritual journey of love, loss, and renewal*. New York: Wiley.

Morrison, R. S., Pewrod, J. D., Cassel, J. B., et al. (2008). Cost savings associated with United States hospital palliative care consultation programs. *Archives of Internal Medicine, 168*(16), 1783–1790.

National Hospice and Palliative Care Organization (NHPCO). (2010). *NHPCO facts and figures: Hospice care in America* (2010 Edn.). Alexandria: NHPCO.

National Institute on Aging. (2008). *End of life: Helping with comfort and care*. Bethesda: National Institutes of Health, U.S. Department of Health and Human Services, NIH Publication No. 08-6036, January.

National Institutes of Health. (2006). *National Institutes of Health State-of-the-Science Conference: Statement on improving end-of-life care*. December 6–8, November 4, 2006. http://consensus.nih.gov/2004/2004EndOfLifeCareSOS024html.htm. Accessed 28 March 2006.

Neufeld, M. J. (1998). Men as caregivers: Reciprocal relationships. *Journal of Advanced Nursing, 28*(5), 959–968.

Nuland, S. B. (1993). *How we die: Reflections on life's final chapter*. New York: Alfred Knopf, Inc.

Rabow, M. W., Hauser, J. M., & Adams, J. (2004). Supporting family caregivers at the end of life "They don't know what they don't know.". *Journal of the American Medical Association, 291*(4), 483–491.

Russell, R. (2001). In sickness and in health: A qualitative study of elderly men who care for their wives with dementia. *Journal of Aging Studies, 15,* 351–367.

Sanders, S., & Power, J. (2009). Roles, responsibilities, and relationships among older husbands caring for wives with progressive dementia and other chronic conditions. *Health & Social Work, 14*(1), 41–51.

Schulz, R., Mendelsohn, A. B., Haley, W. E., Mahoney, D., Allen, R. S., Zhang, S., Thompson, L., & Belle, S. H. (2003). End-of-life care and the effects of bereavement on family caregivers of persons with dementia. *New England Journal of Medicine, 349,* 1936–1942.

Strom, K. M. (2000). *A caregiver's survival guide: How to stay healthy when your loved one is sick*. Downers Grove: Intervarsity Press.

Tada, Y., MacCallum, R. G., McGuire, L., & Kiecolt-Glaser, J. K. (2001). Long-term caregiving: What happens when it ends? *Journal of Abnormal Psychology, 110*(4), 573–584.

Ternel, J. S., Greer, J. A., Muzinkansky, A., et al. (2010). Early palliative care for patients with metastatic non-small cell lung cancer. *New England Journal of Medicine, 363*(8), 733–742.

USA Inc. (2011). *A basic summary of America's financial statements*. February, 2011. www.kcpb.com/usinc or www.amazon.com. Accessed 8 July 2011.

Virnig, B. A., McBean, M., Kind, S., & Rishi, B. A. (2002). Hospice use before death: Variability among cancer diagnoses. *Medical Care, 40*(1), 73–78.

Watson, S. (2010). The forgotten man: Men as caregivers. *Momentum, Fall,* 58–59.

Wayne, M., Robinson, L., & Segal, J. (2012). *End stage and end-of-life care: Caregiving in the final stages of life*. http://www.helpguide.org/elder/alzheimers_disease_dementia_caring_final-stage.htm. Accessed 4 May 2012

Webb, M. (1997). *The good death: The new American search to reshape the end of life*. New York: Bantam Books.

Weitzen, S., Teno, J. M., Fennell, M., et al. (2003). Factors associated with site of death: A national study of where people die. *Medical Care, 41,* 323–335.

Zhang, B., Nilsson, M. E., & Prigerson, H. G. (2012). Factors important to patients' quality of life at the end of life. *Archives of Internal Medicine, 172*(15), 1133–1142.

Zhang, B., Wright, A. A., Huskamp, H. A., Nilsson, M. S., Maciejewski, M. L., Earle, C. C., Block, S. D., Maciejewski, P. K., & Prigerson, H. G. (2009). Health care costs in the last week of life: Associations with conversations. *Archives of Internal Medicine, 169*(5), 480–488.

Chapter 11
The Health of Caregivers

11.1 Introduction

Caregivers have been called “a population at risk” (Family Caregiver Alliance 2012). Evidence shows that most of the estimated 44 million Americans age 18 and older who provide unpaid assistance and support to older people and adults with disabilities and who live in the community are ill-prepared for their role and provide care with little or no support. Nonetheless, one-third of caregivers continue to provide care to others while coping with their own health problems. The Commonwealth Fund Biennial Health Insurance Survey of 2003 found that three-fifths of caregivers reported fair or poor health status, one or more chronic conditions, or a disability, compared to one-third of non-caregivers. Caregivers reported chronic conditions at nearly twice the rate of non-caregivers (see Fig. 11.1). Indeed it is often the worsening of a caregivers own health that influences the decision to place an impaired relative in a long-term care facility if this is a financially and logistically viable option (Navaie-Waliser et al. 2002; Buhr et al. 2006; Whitlatch et al. 1997, 1999; Lieberman and Kramer 1991). Many caregivers especially those with a low income and with tenuous workforce connections are financially vulnerable and lack health insurance which limits access to health care for themselves (Ho et al. 2005). Caregiving is another financial responsibility. The extent to which it becomes a burden depends on a caregiver’s personal and financial resources, their family’s willingness to help, and the use of a support system including respite (Levine 2004).

11.1.1 Caregiving as a Job

There is little debate that the role of caregiver, whether full-time or part-time, is another job, often with new responsibilities and skills acquired on short-notice. If the care recipient is a close family member, the emotional burden may be especially difficult. Caregivers may not be aware of, or deny, the link between the demands of caregiving and its effects on them; there are both positive and negative effects and

J. G. Bruhn, H. M. Rebach, *The Sociology of Caregiving*,
Clinical Sociology: Research and Practice, DOI 10.1007/978-94-017-8857-1_11,

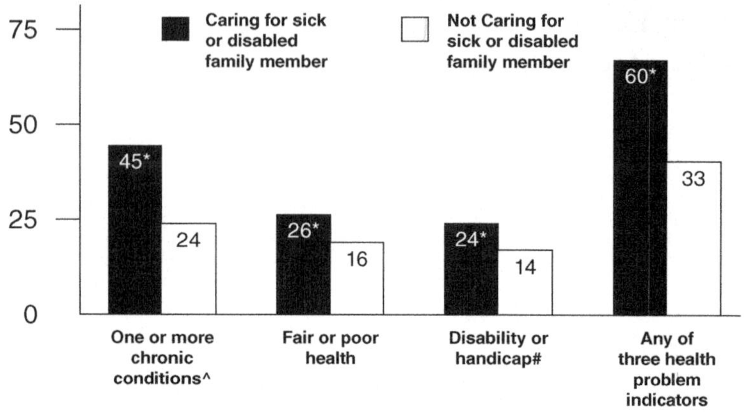

* Significant difference at p≤ .01 or better.

^ Chronic conditions include heart attack/diease, cancer, diabetes or arthritis.

Disability, handicap or chronic disease that prevented full participation in daily work, housework or other daily activities.

Fig. 11.1 Caregivers are more likely than non-caregivers to have health problems. (Source: CDC, National Center for Health Statistics. National Health Interview Survey 2006)

they are cumulative.[1] The degree to which caregivers' own health is at risk depends on their coping skills. The effects of the experience of caregiving are unique to the caregiver and to the care-recipient, and their interaction.

11.1.2 Caregivers' Coping and the Positive and Negative Effects of Caregiving

A frequently used and well-researched model for understanding coping is that proposed by Lazarus and Folkman (1984). They define coping as *constantly changing cognitive and behavioral efforts to manage specific external and/or internal demands that are appraised as taxing or exceeding the resources of the person.* Coping can be focused around problem-solving, emotion, or dealing with social and environmental demands. Coping is a process influenced by personal and situational

[1] The Gallup-Healthways Well-Being Index, established in 2008, surveys the health and well-being of 1,000 Americans by telephone each day. A part of these data relate to caregiver well-being. A February 4, 2011 report indicated that Americans who work a full-time job and say they care for an elderly or disabled family member or relative, suffer from poorer physical health than those who work a full-time job but who do not have additional caregiving responsibilities. The act of caregiving brings with it reduced energy and productivity. Caregivers in all age groups are more likely than non-caregivers to report that poor health keeps them from performing their usual activities and that they did not feel rested the next day. Although specific tasks differ from situation to situation, caregiving often requires more physical activity than normal, which may take a toll on the physical health of caregivers. See well-being index.com.

factors. This transactional view of coping can be applied to the dynamic relationship between caregivers and care-recipients; both need to cope with change as they appraise it and both call upon their resources and experiences in adapting to it. What is stressful, and its degree, depends upon the caregiver's and care-recipient's evaluations of each other and the situation before them. The extent to which the caregiver feels burdened by the care-recipient has been shown to be a significant factor in their mutual well-being. Caregivers attributed to the recipients affective levels similar to their own (Schulz et al. 1987).

Not all change or stress is negative or maladaptive; people can learn from stress and apply their learning both cognitively and emotionally to new situations. What is key in Lazarus and Folkman's model is to develop and use coping processes that result in an adaptational outcome, that is, levels of health, morale and social functioning that are appropriate for the recipient. The caregiver helps the recipient to fulfill his or her roles appropriate to their state of health. When the boundaries between the caregiver's health and well-being and the care-recipient's needs and demands become blurred or unrealistic, the relationship encounters frequent conflict and poor outcomes. This is a greater possibility when the dependence of a needy person becomes absolute (Kass 2005; Kane and West 2004).

11.1.3 Multiple Roles

Kass (2005) pointed out that caregivers are not caregivers *only*. They can occupy multiple roles which they can hold simultaneously. Multiple roles can be associated with both positive and negative consequences (Stephens et al. 1994; Jenkins 1997). Some evidence suggests that multiple roles provide opportunities and advantages. Coser (1975) argued that multiple roles enable individuals to express their individuality and therefore are important for the development of personality and intellect. It has been found that women who hold many roles have better health than women holding only a few roles (Verbrugge 1983). Furthermore, role sharing can outweigh potential negative consequences of multiple roles. There is evidence that benefits are associated with multiple roles that may help to offset some of the stress. For example, caregivers who are able to participate in and perform a number of different roles experience not only less role strain but also lower rates of depression and wider self-esteem (Marks and MacDermid 1996). Benefits and stress can balance each other, and it is the accumulation of one or the other that most affects the caregiver's well-being (Franks and Stephens 1996).

Whether multiple roles benefit or harm women's health depends upon how women actively manage role combinations (Pavalko and Woodbury 2000) and manage the meaning that giving care provides them (Kim et al. 2006). Even when caregiving demands become intense, caregivers often cite positive aspects of the experience. They report that caregiving makes them feel good about themselves, gives meaning to their lives, enables them to learn new skills, and strengthens their relationships with others (Tarlow et al. 2004).[2] Indeed, it has been found that mortality was significantly reduced for individuals who reported giving instrumental support to their friends, relatives and neighbors and who provided emotional support to their spouse (Brown et al. 2003). We need to learn how social support and resources and caregiving mastery, (Kim and Kim 2005) moderate the stressful aspects of caregiving (Schulz and Sherwood 2008).[3]

11.2 Social Support as a Moderator of Caregiving Stress

According to Vitaliano et al. (2003), caring for a family member with dementia is regarded as a chronically stressful process with potentially negative physical health consequences. Yet, they did not find quantitative studies that tested this hypothesis. They searched the literature over a 38 year period and found only 23 studies that compared physical health indicators in family caregivers with demographically similar noncaregivers. While they found that caregivers had a 23 % higher level of stress hormones and a 15 % lower level of antibody responses than did noncaregivers, these observational data did not permit them to make inferences that caregiving is hazardous to one's health. Rather than looking for "causes" of caregiving illness, Vitaliano and his colleagues suggest that a broader perspective of the health effects of caregiving should frame future studies and include various chronic diseases and various age groups of caregivers with different comorbidities for the risk for health problems in response to stress.

Certainly caregiving is more or less stressful for both caregivers and care-recipients at different times during the process of caregiving. Aneshensel et al. (1995) have referred to caregiving an as unexpected career because caregiving is analogous to executing a career in a number of ways: (1) it encompasses a role and its consequences; (2) it conveys a sense of movement and change; and (3) it is more or less structured. That does not mean that caregiving is a universal process followed by all caregivers, indeed variations in coping make much of caregiving situationally and personally unique. Caregiving, therefore, is not stressful in the same way or to the same degree for all caregivers. Much, if not all of stress is interactional, rising out of social situations conducive to stress, especially situations relating to boundary transactions. Also the interaction between the coping styles of caregivers and care recipients creates situations conducive to stress. How caregivers cope with

[2] S. B. Hudnall believes that compassion satisfaction reduces the negative effects of compassion fatigue. He developed a compassion satisfaction scale to identify the positive effects of caregiving in an effort to understand the relationship between the positive and negative aspects of compassion. See S. B. Hudnall, Measuring compassion satisfaction as well as fatigue. Developmental history of the compassion satisfaction and fatigue test. In Figley (1995).

[3] For detailed information and data on Seniors and Caregivers see the results of the online survey conducted by Harris Interactive on behalf of the American Academy of Family Physicians in March, 2012 http://www.sacbee.com/2012/04/24/4438303/caregiving-affects-health-of-three.html. Also see the National Alliance for Caregiving & Evercare (2006).

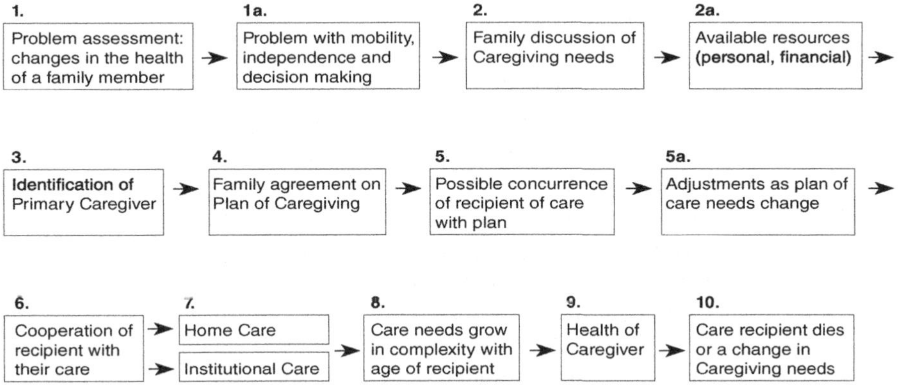

Fig. 11.2 Key steps in decision making in the evolution of caregiving

situations conducive to stress is key to understanding why some caregivers emerge from a caregiving career with health problems. Individuals confront the stressors in caregiving much like they confront other stressors in their lives, that is, how they moderate stress to minimize its adverse effects. It is our belief that caregivers who have available strong support resources, and use them, are less likely to be overwhelmed by singular or accumulated episodes of stress in caregiving.

11.3 The Roles, Dynamics, and Outcomes of Caregiving and Receiving

Aneshensel et al. (1995) use dementia to describe the process of caregiving as it progresses through three stages or pathways: (1) role acquisition; (2) role enactment; and (3) role disengagement paralleling three major transitions in dementia caregiving: (1) illness onset; (2) nursing home admission; and (3) death of the patient. While the transitional conceptualization is useful, and most of caregiving research to date has focused on dementia, we do not believe this conceptualization is generalizable to non-dementia illnesses that do not require institutionalization or all types of informal caregiving. Also, the Aneshensel's model is linear and therefore, limited (p. 24). Vachon (1999) pointed out that a circular conceptualization of the process of caregiving is more appropriate because cycling is an expected part of illness progression.We benefitted from Aneshensel's idea of caregiving as a career although we have named the phases of the progression of the caregiving role differently, i.e. role initiation, role performance, and role completion. We have also adopted Vachon's idea of caregiving as a circular process, conveying that it is dynamic, interactive, and cumulative. Figure 11.2 is provided to help understand the roles, dynamics and outcomes of caregiving and receiving.

11.3.1 Role Initiation

Caregiving begins in the family with concern over a change in a member's ability to function physically, psychologically and/or emotionally. The family may wish to visit a physician for evaluation of the family member. The outcome of this visit can be home care, assisted living, nursing home care, or other facility with supervision. The family may have a conference to discuss these care alternatives with or without the care recipient's input. The place of care is often determined by whether the proposed recipient lives alone, with a spouse, or with family or relatives and their ability to perform required activities of daily living. Age, health status, level of functioning and financial resources are the key elements influencing where caregiving will be provided and by whom. Sometimes families have the resources, but lack the motivation, energy, and commitment to provide caregiving themselves and the proposed recipient is placed in a facility for care to be given by formal caregivers.

The extent of the family support system is very important in the assessment of the need for caregiving. In considering possible caregivers in the family it has been typical to look for female adults. However, young emerging adult caregivers aged 18–25 years, including men, are beginning to be recognized as a growing subpopulation (Levine et al. 2005). These young adults who are caregivers now are only the first wave of future caregivers. It is speculated that in the future, with delayed childbearing and smaller families, aging parents will have to look to young men and women under age 25 who are still in their formative years for help. Often if a family member volunteers to be the major caregiver the rest of the family withdraws from caregiving; at the other extreme, especially in cultures that are family-oriented, the entire family is supportive and participates in caregiving in some way.

What is troublesome is when family members literally abandon a member needing care to a facility. While geographic separation and job requirements, such as frequent travel, complicate family's participation in caregiving, it can lead to "forgetting" about the member who is remembered by a card on special holidays. There are real constraints such as age (too young or too old) and poor health that prohibit family members who want to be a caregiver but can't. Sometimes, however, a family member may become a caregiver for another member by default. The nature of a family's support system is a good predictor of the degree of satisfaction a care giver and recipient have in their care experience as well as the recipient's longevity.

11.3.2 Role Performance

a. *The Caregiver*

   Several factors influence the effectiveness of a caregiver's role performance. *First*, does the identified caregiver have the skills and degree of objectivity to perform as a caregiver? If the identified caregiver is too emotionally invested in the care recipient's condition, the caregiver may not be able to make appropriate decisions and not have the necessary stamina to cope with the ups and downs of a progressive condition.[4] *Second*, if the identified caregiver is engaged in multiple roles, including caretaking for another family member, the physical and emotional load may require a degree of additional help from volunteers, friends or family. Even caregivers with good coping skills need respite and support. *Third*, the caregiver's role performance is influenced by the duration and intensity of care required by the care recipient's condition. A severely disabled and dependent care recipient will require constant vigilance by the caregiver 24 h a day. The demands for care come from both the condition and the personality of the recipient, and their variability. *Fourth*, it requires a healthy caregiver to provide consistent, positive, high quality caregiving. The effects of the demands of caregiving on the health of caregivers are short-term and long-term. Schulz and Tompkins (2010) pointed out that the tasks of caregiving are cumulative, often become more complex, and intensive. Therefore, caregiving needs may exceed a caregiver's skills. This may require the caregiver to obtain additional skills or additional help.

b. *The Care Recipient*
   How well a caregiver performs their role is also related to the degree to which the care recipient accepts their role and acts cooperatively. Personality conflicts can exacerbate the symptoms of a condition and complicate caregiving for both the giver and recipient. The stress of caregiving and receiving needs to have an outlet and the options for releasing stress may be conflicts expressed as impatience, forms of disrespect or even physical or psychological abuse. The stress of care receiving may be apparent when the recipient acts depressed and either has no living family or family who provide little or no social support for the recipient. The level of a care recipient's dependency is usually a good indicator of possible frustration and anger, especially if the recipient occupies their time with sleeping and/or television. It is not surprising to find care recipients who are highly dependent on others for assistance and yet express feelings of depression, aggression, and giving up.

Newsom and Schulz (1998) identified predictors of negative reactions to assistance provided to a physically disabled spouse and the consequences that negative reactions have for the mental health of the care recipient. Nearly 40 % of care recipients reported some emotional distress in response to help they received. Fatalistic attitudes, perceived control, and low self-esteem predicted greater helping distress, whereas low self-esteem, fatalistic beliefs and marital conflict were likely to lead to helping distress for those who received high levels of assistance. Helping distress was found to predict depression as long as 1 year later, suggesting that there may be long-term consequences of negative reactions to assistance. Therefore, it is possible that a cycle of negative behavior can emerge between caregiver/care recipient marital pairs over time as the care recipient's condition worsens (Beach et al. 2000).

[4] See the excellent article by Wilber (1988). Wilber discusses the trials and tribulations of being a primary support person for his wife who had cancer.

There are care recipients who are accepting of their condition and situation and act cooperatively and express appreciation for their care; this attitude and behavior impacts positively on the caregiver's ability to perform their role with optimism and satisfaction as well.

11.3.3 Role Outcomes

a. For Caregivers
   The possible role outcomes for a primary caregiver can be: (1) complete the role of caregiver with satisfaction and no apparent health effects; (2) complete the role of caregiver with mixed emotions and negative health effects; and (3) modify the role of primary caregiver to a shared or supportive one.
   Family culture has a significant effect on the outcome of caregiving roles (Pinquart and Sorensen 2005). Cultures that are family-oriented and have a high degree of social cohesion, shared roles and responsibilities, and commonly-held belief systems view caregiving as a part of family life. For example, there is a strong cultural norm among Hispanics that women provide care to dependent elders; among Asian Americans, the oldest son and his wife are expected to take the caregiver role; and African-American female caregivers select adult children and other relatives to help with caregiving (Lehman 2009). Institutionalization does occur, but as a last resort. It has been found that caregivers who institutionalize their relatives are more likely to become bereaved than those whose relatives continue to reside in the home or community (Aneshensel et al. 1995). A strong cultural commitment keeps caregiving from becoming a burden on any one family member. One would expect that such a cultural commitment would protect against adverse health effects for caregivers.
b. For Care Recipients
   Care recipients can experience several different outcomes. Of course gradual decline and death is one. The recipient may be rehabilitated and recover. The recipient's dependency may worsen making it necessary to transfer to a formal care facility. Nursing home patients have been found to die sooner than patients who remain at home (Aneshensel et al. 1995). Some services, such as hospice care, can be provided in the home. The context of care can greatly influence the care recipient's attitude and hopefulness. A recipient of hospice care may "improve" to the extent that it is necessary to take the person off of hospice services, only to return when his/her condition worsens.

Caregiving quality has important health effects for the care recipient. The caregiver who maintains good psychological and physical health, who does not feel burdened by caregiving, and who has a sense of self efficacy will likely provide better care than one who has deficits in these areas. The degree that caregiving is supportive to the care of the recipient without promoting dependency or being critical, there will be an optimum environment providing positive health effects for the recipient (Vachon 1999).

11.4 Predicting Caregiver Health Effects and Mortality

Predicting caregivers' health and mortality is difficult to do because we can't assume caregivers' health status, favorable or unfavorable, is attributable solely to the caregiver role. Also, caregivers may not be fully aware of, deny, or minimize their state of health prior to becoming a caregiver. The symptoms of some diseases are subtle, variable, slowly progressive and not part of our daily awareness. Furthermore, caregivers engage in other roles and life activities that are intertwined with caregiving so cause and effect for any one event or role is confounded. Finally, evidence of caregivers' health is often not documented except by memory. And, still, some caregivers may not experience health effects until after the recipient's death.[5,6] Therefore, the need for longitudinal studies using comparison or control groups is essential if research findings are to be replicated, generalized and interventions planned. We will confine our discussion of caregiver health effects and mortality to longitudinal studies (Montgomery 1996).

11.4.1 Health Effects

The Caregiver Health Effects Study (CHES) is an ancillary study of the Cardiovascular Health Study (CHS), a large prospective population-based cohort of approximately 400 elderly spousal caregivers and 400 age and sex matched noncaregivers followed for a period of 4 years by researchers at the University of Pittsburgh (Schulz and Beach 1999). Results suggest that caring for a disabled spouse is a stressful experience with possible negative consequences, but at the same time caregivers may derive some mental health benefits from helping a spouse in need (Beach et al. 2000). The largest negative effects observed among caregivers were those who characterized themselves as being strained (Schulz et al. 1997). Caregivers with compromised mental and physical health were more likely to provide lower quality care to the recipient but also be at high risk for engaging in harmful behavior toward them (Beach et al. 2005). Caregivers providing long hours of care over extended time periods had raised levels of distress; in women more than men. Adverse effects on caregivers such as depression have been found to be prevalent

[5] Studies of caregiver health effects are difficult to summarize or compare because of methodological issues. There is great variance in the caregiving experience of persons classified as caregivers providing care to persons with a wide range of disabilities and a wide range of intensity and frequency of caregiving demands. Some study designs are cross-sectional, others are longitudinal; some samples are small and unrepresentative; some define and assess caregiving differently; some only look at negative effects; some do not have comparison groups; some have uncontrolled confounding effects. Evaluating longitudinal studies is complicated by differences in the number and spacing of follow-up interviews, and lack baseline measures before caregiving begins. See Baumgarten (1989).

[6] See McLeod (1999). A powerful book of stories and practical action steps from an author caring for aging parents, one with ALS and dementia.

around transitioning points in care; e.g. the beginning and end of care (Hirst 2005; Marks et al. 2002).

The effects of helping appear to depend strongly on the nature of the relationship between the caregiver and care recipient (Poulin et al. 2010). The benefits of helping are enhanced and the costs minimized when there is a strong sense of interdependence between the caregiver and those who are cared for. Although prior caregiving research has linked being a caregiver primarily with negative outcomes, recent research using a longitudinal design suggests that providing full-time home care predicts better health and even reduced mortality among spouse caregivers (Brown et al. 2009). The time spent giving care predicted greater levels of positive affect and this association was greater among caregivers who perceived themselves as interdependent with the care recipient (their spouse).

Longitudinal studies have found that changes in the care recipient's health were not predictive of caregivers' physical or mental health (Goode et al. 1998). Rather caregivers who report the greatest increase in physical symptoms were those who had low initial social support. Psychosocial resource variables (appraisals, coping responses, and social support) do predict longitudinal changes in caregiver mental and physical health (Goode et al. 1998). Caregivers with lower social support and less personal control perceived their caregiving role as more burdensome and less rewarding than did caregivers with high social support and more personal control (Hwang et al. 2011).

Research findings suggest that the positive aspects of caregiving are mainly related to specific characteristics of caregivers, i.e. being a caregiver by one's own initiative, with maintaining leisure time, with less use of ventive emotions, with the caregiver not working out of home, and with previous affectionate relationships between the caregiver and care recipient (Lopez et al. 2005). A need for time away from the recipient was found to be a major quality of life concern for highly burdened caregivers (Coen et al. 2002).

11.4.2 Mortality

Caregivers who report strain associated with caregiving are more likely to die than noncaregiving controls (Schulz and Beach 1999). This finding is consistent with other outcomes for the University of Pittsburgh cohort showing that strained caregivers compared with matched noncaregiving controls have significantly higher levels of depression and anxiety, and lower levels of perceived health. They are also less likely to get enough rest, have time to rest when they are sick, or have time to exercise. All of these factors, and others, are possible mediators between caregiving and mortality (Schulz and Beach 1999). Caregiver strain and hospitalization of the spouse has been linked to increased caregiver mortality risk (Christakis and Allison 2009). Yet, Brown et al. (2009) found that spending at least 14 h per week providing care to their spouse predicted decreased mortality for the caregiver. It may be premature to conclude that health risks for caregivers are due to providing help. Under some circumstances caregivers may benefit from providing care (Brown et al. 2009). This suggests a paradox, namely that helping other people can be both bad and good for one's health. Moderation or effective coping and the ability to take care of one's self may control the negative effects or lighten the burden of caregiving. Of course, the nature of the recipient's illness and the degree of support available to the caregiver are also mediating effects for caregiver mortality. A recent study found that, although caregivers report stress those that are more physically active seem to be protected from health decline (Fredman et al. 2008).

11.5 The Quality of the Caregiver-Recipient Relationship as a Predictor of Caregiver and Recipient Health

Family members have high expectations of the care given to their ill, aged, or disabled loved one irrespective of whether they are directly involved in that care or not. Caregiving is expected, especially when given by a family member, to be nurturing and reciprocal. Family members sometimes believe that age and illness are timeless and surmise more stability than realistic. Their communal relationship is subject to change. Caregivers can become compromised mentally and/or physically and provide lower quality care which can lead over time to abuse or neglect, and ultimately to negative health outcomes for the care recipient (Beach et al. 2005). Yet, change, while a predictable factor that can alter a nurturing, and reciprocal relationship, often has unpredictable effects. One of the attributes of excellent caregiving is for the caregivers themselves to cope with changes in the aging and disease processes and assist the recipient to do so as well. A sudden heart attack, stroke, or fall can change a recipient's mobility and/or cognitive functions, limiting or eliminating verbal communication and altering reciprocity between giver and receiver. Communal orientation and closeness of the caregiver-recipient relationship has been studied as predictors of distress among caregivers of Alzheimer's patients. Caregivers perceived caregiving as less stressful when they felt high levels of affection for the care recipient. Similarly, caregivers who received more rewards from their care recipients experienced lower levels of burden (Williamson et al. 2001). Therefore, it is not surprising that change in the caregiver-recipient relationship was found to be associated with high levels of depression (Williamson and Schulz 1990). When caregivers were at risk for clinical depression care recipients were more likely to report that their caregiver screamed and yelled at them, called them names, or swore at them (Beach et al. 2005).

Changes in the caregiving-care receiving relationship may alter the effects of helping (Poulin et al. 2010). The transition to a caregiving relationship is frequently marked by a loss of reciprocity between relationship partners, making acts of helping feel more burdensome for the caregiver.

11.6 Summary

Caregiving can be a job itself, especially as people live longer and experience the downside of aging, chronic disease and disability requiring part-time or full-time help. Indeed, caregiving has been called a career. Caregiving can be stressful for the care recipient depending upon the state of health of the recipient and the resources available to them, and for the caregiver depending upon their coping skills, state of health, support and assistance from others, and the intensity and duration of the caregiving situation. There are many cross-sectional studies and testimonials describing the negative effects that caregiving can have on a caregiver's health and longevity. There are few studies on the positive effects of caregiving on caregiver's health and well-being. Since there are many factors that can be in play during the process of caregiving there is a need for more longitudinal studies with comparison groups that more vigorously control for confounding variables. For example, we need to know how social support moderates the stressful aspects of caregiving. We proposed a circular conceptualization of the process of caregiving to convey its continued interactive aspects from role initiation to role completion.

Researchers are interested in predicting caregiver's health and mortality so that appropriate stress-reducing interventions can be planned and implemented. Caregivers with compromised mental and physical health are more likely to provide lower quality care to a recipient and also be at high risk for engaging in harmful behavior toward them. The effects of a helping relationship are enhanced and the costs minimized when there is a strong sense of interdependence between the caregiver and the recipient. Research findings suggest that the positive aspects of caregiving are mainly related to specific characteristics of caregivers such as being a caregiver by one's own initiative, with maintaining leisure time, and less use of ventive emotions. A need for respite for the recipient has been found to be a major quality of life concern for highly burdened caregivers.

11.7 Questions for Discussion

1. Discuss the positive aspects of caregiving and how they can overcome the negative aspects.
2. How does social support work as a moderator of caregiving stress?
3. What is meant by caregiving as a career?
4. Explain the process of role initiation, role performance, and role outcomes.
5. What is the state of our knowledge in predicting caregiver health effects? Discuss.
6. Discuss differences in the roles of informal and formal caregiving.

References

Aneshensel, C. S., Pearlin, L. I., Mullan, J. T., Zarit, S. H., & Whitlatch, C. J. (1995). *Profiles in caregiving: The unexpected career*. New York: Academic Press.

Baumgarten, M. (1989). The health of persons giving care to the demented elderly: A critical review of the literature. *Journal of Clinical Epidemiology, 42,* 1137–1148.

Beach, S. R., Schulz, R., Yee, J. L., & Jackson, S. (2000). Negative and positive health effects of caring for a disabled spouse: Longitudinal findings from the caregiver health effects study. *Psychology & Aging, 15*(2), 259–271.

Beach, S. R., Schulz, R., Williamson, G. M., Miller, L. S., Weiner, M. F., & Lance, C. E. (2005). Risk factors for potentially harmful informal caregiver behavior. *Journal of the American Geriatrics Society, 53,* 255–261.

Brown, S. L., Nesse, R. M., Vinokur, A. D., & Smith, D. M. (2003). Providing social support may be more beneficial than receiving it: Results from a prospective study of mortality. *Psychological Science, 14*(4), 320–327.

Brown, S. L., Smith, D. M., Schulz, R., Kabeto, M. U., Ubel, P. A., Poulin, M. J., & Langa, K. M. (2009). Caregiving behavior is associated with decreased mortality risk. *Psychological Science, 20,* 488–494.

Buhr, G. T., Kuchibhatia, M., & Clipp, E. (2006). Caregivers' reasons for nursing home placement: Cues for improving discussions with families prior to the transition. *The Gerontologist, 46*(1), 52–61.

Christakis, N. A., & Allison, P. D. (2009). Inter-spousal mortality effects caregiver burden across the spectrum of disabling disease. In D. M. Cutler & D. A. Wise (Eds.), *Health at older ages: The causes and consequences of declining disability among the elderly* (pp. 455–477). Chicago: University of Chicago Press.

Coen, R. F., O'Boyle, C. A., Coakley, D., & Lawlor, B. A. (2002). Individual quality of life factors distinguishing low-burden and high-burden caregivers of dementia patients. *Dementia and Geriatric Cognitive Disorders, 13*(3), 164–170.

Commonwealth Fund Biennial Health Insurance Survey. (2003). http://www.commonwealthfund.org/Search.aspx?search=caregiver+health+problem&Filefilter=1. Accessed 1 July 2012.

Coser, R. L. (1975). The complexity of roles as a seed bed of individual autonomy. In L. Coser (Ed.), *The idea of social structure* (pp. 237–263). New York: Harcourt.

Family Caregiver Alliance Website. (2012). http://www.caregiver.org/caregiver/jsp/content_node.jsp?nodeid=1822. Accessed 8 June 2013.

Figley, C. R. (Ed.). (1995). *Treating compassion fatigue. Psychosocial stress series, no. 24* (pp. 107–119). New York: Brunner-Routledge.

Franks, M. M., & Stephens, M. A. P. (1996). Social support in the context of caregiving: Husbands' provision of support to wives involved in patient care. *Journals of Gerontology: Psychological Sciences, 51B,* P43–P52.

Fredman, L., Cauley, J. A., Satterfield, S., Simonsick, E., Spencer, M., Ayonayon, H. N., & Harris, T. B. (2008). Caregiving, mortality, and mobility decline: The health, aging, and body composition (Health ABC) study. *Archives of Internal Medicine, 168*(19), 2154–2162.

Goode, K. T., Haley, W. E., Roth, D. L., & Ford, G. (1998). Predicting longitudinal changes in caregiver physical and mental health: A stress process model. *Health Psychology, 17*(2), 190–198.

Hirst, M. (2005). Carer distress: A prospective, population-based study. *Social Science & Medicine, 61,* 697–708.

Ho, A., Collins, S. R., Davis, K., & Doty, M. M. (2005). *A look at working-age caregivers' roles, health concerns, and need for support.* The Commonwealth Fund Issue Brief #854, August. Washington, DC.

Hwang, B., Fleischmann, K. E., Howie-Esquivel, J., Stotts, N. A., & Dracup, K. (2011). Caregiving for patients with heart failure: Impact on patients' families. *American Journal of Critical Care, 20*(6), 431–441.

Jenkins, J. L. (1997). Women, work, and caregiving: How do these roles affect women's well-being? *Journal of Women & Aging, 9*(3), 27–45.
Kane, R. L., & West, J. G. (2004). Pushing the boundaries in assisted living: Failures in caring. In C. Levine (Ed.), *Always on call: When illness turns families into caregivers* (pp. 54–65). Nashville: Vanderbilt University Press.
Kass, L. R. (2005). *Taking care: Ethical caregiving in our aging society*. Washington, DC: The President's Council on Bioethics.
Kim, J. H., & Kim, O. S. (2005). Influencing factors that affect the psychological well-being in family caregivers of stroke patients. *Taehan Kanho Hakhoe Chu, 35*(2), 399–406.
Kim, Y., Baker, F., Spillers, R. L., & Wellisch, D. K. (2006). Psychological adjustment of cancer caregivers with multiple roles. *Psycho-Oncology, 15*(9), 795–804.
Lazarus, R. S., & Folkman, S. (1984). *Stress, appraisal, and coping*. New York: Springer.
Lehman, D. (2009). 21st century caregivers: Diversity in culture. *Aging Well*, 2, 26. http://www.agingwellmag.com/archive/030209p26.shtml. Accessed 20 June 2012.
Levine, C. (2004). The loneliness of the long-term caregiver. In C. Levine (Ed.), *Always on call: When illness turns families into caregivers* (pp. 99–107). Nashville: Vanderbilt University Press.
Levine, C., Gibson, G., Halper, D., Hart, A. Y., Lautz, J., & Gould, D. A. (2005). Young adult caregivers: A first look at an unstudied population. *American Journal of Public Health, 95*(11), 2071–2075.
Lieberman, M. A., & Kramer, J. H. (1991). Factors affecting decisions to institutionalize demented elderly. *The Gerontologist, 31*(3), 371–374.
Lopez, J., Lopez-Arrieta, J., & Crespo, M. (2005). Factors associated with the positive impact of caring for elderly and dependent relatives. *Archives of Gerontology & Geriatrics, 41,* 81–94.
Marks, N. F., Lambert, J. D., & Choi, H. (2002). Transitions to caregiving, gender, and psychological well-being: A prospective U.S. National Study. *Journal of Marriage & Family, 64*(August), 657–667.
Marks, S. R., & MacDermid, S. M. (1996). Multiple roles and the self: A theory of role balance. *Journal of Marriage and the Family, 58,* 417–432.
McLeod, B. W. (1999). *Caregiving: The spiritual journey of love, loss, and renewal*. New York: Wiley.
Montgomery, R. J. V. (1996). Advancing caregiver research: Weighing efficacy and feasibility of interventions. *The Journals of Gerontology: Series B, 51B*(3), S109–S110.
National Alliance for Caregiving & Evercare. (2006). *Evercare study of caregivers in decline: A close-up look at the health risks of caring for a loved one*. Bethesda: National Alliance for Caregiving and Minnetonka, MN: Evercare.
Navaie-Waliser, M., Feldman, P. H., Gould, D. A., Levine, C. L., Kuerbis, A. N., & Donelan, K. (2002). When the caregiver needs care: The plight of vulnerable caregivers. *American Journal of Public Health, 92*(3), 409–413.
Newsom, J. T., & Schulz, R. (1998). Caregiving from the recipient's perspective: Negative reactions to being helped. *Health Psychology, 17*(2), 172–181.
Pavalko, E. K., & Woodbury, S. (2000). Social roles as process: Caregiving careers and women's health. *Journal of Health and Social Behavior, 41*(1), 91–105.
Pinquart, M., & Sorensen, S. (2005). Ethnic differences in stressors, resources, and psychological outcomes of family caregiving: A meta-analysis. *The Gerontologist, 45*(1), 90–106.
Poulin, M. J., Brown, S. L., Ubel, P. A., Smith, D. A., Jankovic, A., & Langa, K. M. (2010). Does a helping hand mean a heavy heart? Helping behavior and well-being among spouse caregivers. *Psychological Aging, 25*(1), 108–117.
Schulz, R., & Beach, S. R. (1999). Caregiving as a risk factor for mortality. *Journal of the American Medical Association, 282*(23), 2215–2219.
Schulz, R., & Sherwood, P. R. (2008). Physical and mental health effects of family caregiving. *Journal of Social Work Education, 44*(3), 105–113.
Schulz, R., & Tompkins, C. A. (2010). Informal caregivers in the United States: Prevalence, caregiver characteristics, and ability to provide care. In S. Olson (Ed.), *The role of human factors*

in home health care, workshop summary (pp. 117–143). Washington, DC: The National Academies Press.

Schulz, R., Tompkins, C. A., Wood, D., & Decker, S. (1987). The social psychology of caregiving: Physical and psychological costs of providing support to the disabled. *Journal of Applied Psychology, 17*(4), 401–428.

Schulz, R., Newsom, J., Mittelmark, M., Burton, L., Hirsch, C., & Jackson, S. (1997). Health effects of caregiving: The caregiver health effects study: An ancillary study of the cardiovascular health study. *Annals of Behavioral Medicine, 19*(2), 110–116.

Stephens, M. P., Franks, M. M., & Townsend, A. L. (1994). Stress and rewards in women's multiple roles: The care of women in the middle. *Psychology and Aging, 9*(1), 45–52.

Tarlow, B. J., Wisniewski, S. R., Belle, S. H., Rubert, M., Ory, M. G., & Gallagher-Thompson, D. (2004). Positive aspects of caregiving: Contributions of the REACH Project to the development of new measures for Alzheimer's caregiving. *Research on Aging, 26*(4), 429–480.

Vachon, D. O. (1999). The health effects of caregiving for adults in later life. In T. L. Whitman, T. V. Merluzzi, & R. D. White (Eds.), *Life-span perspectives on health and illness* (pp. 227–248). Mahwah: Lawrence Erlbaum Associates.

Verbrugge, L. (1983). Multiple roles and physical health of women and men. *Journal of Health and Social Behavior, 24,* 16–30.

Vitaliano, P. P., Zang, J., & Scanlan, J. M. (2003). Is caregiving hazardous to one's physical health?: A meta-analysis. *Psychological Bulletin, 129*(6), 946–972.

Whitlatch, C. J., Feinberg, L. F., & Sebasta, D. S. (1997). Depression and health in family caregivers. *Journal of Aging and Health, 9*(2), 222–243.

Whitlatch, C. J., Feinberg, L. F., & Stevens, E. J. (1999). Predictors of institutionalization for persons with Alzheimer's disease and the impact on family caregivers. *Journal of Mental Health and Aging, 5*(3), 275–288.

Wilber, K. (1988). On being a support person. *The Journal of Transpersonal Psychology, 20*(2), 141–159.

Williamson, G. M., & Schulz, R. (1990). Relationship orientation, quality of prior relationship, and distress among caregivers of Alzheimer's patients. *Psychology and Aging, 3*(4), 502–509.

Williamson, G. M., Shaffer, D. R., & The Family Relationships in Late Life Project. (2001). Relationship quality and potentially harmful behaviors by spousal caregivers: How we were then, how we are now. *Psychology and Aging, 16*(2), 217–226.

Chapter 12
Legal and Ethical Issues in Caregiving

12.1 Introduction

"For many health professionals in the United States the concept of respect for autonomy has come to be the principle that trumps all other principles" (Kuczewski and Polansky 2000).[1] The principle of autonomy requires respect for the decision-making capacity of competent adults. Efforts to improve end-of-life decision-making quality have emphasized the principle of individual autonomy to better ensure that patients receive care consistent with their preferences. This principle has been primarily defined through court decisions during the past several decades as a patient's right to refuse medical technologies and avoid life-prolonging treatments. However, autonomy as traditionally defined only serves a small segment of dying patients. Patients might not value autonomy or consider autonomy important, but define it differently than decision-making self-determination. Some also think in terms of their care goals rather than individual treatment preferences. Patients' functional and cognitive abilities, age, racial and ethnic backgrounds, and desire to avoid burdening loved ones may influence attitudes and definitions regarding autonomy (Winzelberg et al. 2005).

Ethical issues near the end of life often arise because of concerns about how much and what kind of care make sense for someone with a limited life expectancy, particularly if the patient is very ill. There is often conflict between health professionals and family members about what constitutes appropriate care. Many conflicts can be avoided by clarifying who makes the difficult decisions to limit care and by advance care planning. Caregivers should begin making legal preparations soon after their loved one has been diagnosed with a serious illness.

In this chapter we discuss the major legal and ethical issues that encompass family caregiving to better understand decision-making burdens on families and how the burden of caregiving can result in various types and levels of caregiver abuse, neglect and exploitation.

[1] See Gessert (2008).

J. G. Bruhn, H. M. Rebach, *The Sociology of Caregiving*,
Clinical Sociology: Research and Practice, DOI 10.1007/978-94-017-8857-1_12,

12.2 Planning for Incapacity: Legal Issues of Caregiving

12.2.1 Decision-Making

The physician, proposed care recipient and proposed caregiver should participate together in medical decision-making. Available data suggest that patients with terminal cancer are more likely to receive end-of-life care that is consistent with their preferences when they have had the opportunity to discuss their wishes with their physician (Mack et al. 2010). However, the incidence of dementia has been found to be substantial among those age 85 and over (14 times higher than those aged 65–69), which usually precludes the understanding of many of the issues involved in choosing among treatment alternatives (Hebert et al. 1995). In addition, many cognitively intact elderly are incapable of complex discussions about their care. In these situations a surrogate must be identified to speak on behalf of the proposed recipient. The physician must access the recipient's decision-making capacity, that is, whether the proposed care recipient is capable of making voluntary, informed, authentic, and autonomous medical choices (Kapp 1991). Decisional capacity is not a global, all-or-nothing matter, but is dependent upon the complexity of the particular decision confronting the person at the time. Decision-making capacity can vary over time and depend on factors such as drugs taken, persons present, physical surroundings, methods of communication used and perceived pressures from those present. One of the main safeguards is to assure that decisions are not overridden by family caregivers with their own agendas and by those formal caregivers who are asked to carry out the family's instructions (Kapp 1991).

The initial conversation that the family has with the proposed care recipient can be either problematic or unchallenging depending upon the proposed care recipient's personality, the effects of illness on them, past history of family problem-solving and current familial relationships, and perceived or real pressure of family members to decide whether or not the proposed recipient of care agrees that a caretaker needs to be identified and the appropriate legal documents need to be completed. While clearly written legal documents that outline the proposed care recipient's wishes are needed to assure that a protocol will be followed in implementing decisions, changing family dynamics, especially as the care recipient's illness progresses, can revive covert family issues as emotions surface. This is why the thoroughness of the decision-making process for advanced directives is so important. Family members should be enablers and supporters of their ill relative and demonstrate that they wish to cooperate in the plan for their relative's incapacity.

After a physician has given input into the medical assessment of the proposed care recipient's degree of autonomy in decision-making about their health, the advice and services of an attorney are needed.[2] If the proposed care recipient is age

[2] Many people think that drafting an advance directive is complicated and expensive and requires a lawyer. However, forms for every state (state laws regarding advance directives differ) are available on the Internet, at the *National Hospice and Palliative Care Organization's Web site* or through the *National Healthcare Decision Day site*. An advance directive only needs a few dollars for the services of a notary.

65 or older, an attorney who practices elder law, a specialized area of law focusing on issues that typically affect older adults can be especially helpful. For those who can't afford a lawyer there are resources to help such as federally funded programs, pro bono programs, self-help clinics, and low-cost legal programs. Some law schools have law clinics staffed by law students and some communities have legal aid services listed in the yellow pages of the telephone book.

12.3 Advance Directives

Advance directives can serve several important values. "They can preserve well-being by protecting the individual from intrusive and futile medical interventions; they can promote self-determination; and they can serve as vehicles for altruism by authorizing termination of treatment that would impose financial and emotional costs on others" (Buchanan and Brock 1989, p. 152).

Advance directives (ADs) are usually written documents designed to allow competent patients the opportunity to guide future healthcare decisions in the event that they are unable to participate in medical decision-making. A federal law, in 1991, the *Patient Self-Determination Act,* requires that patients be informed about their right to participate in health-care decisions, including their right to have an advance directive. Advance directives fall into two broad categories: instructive and proxy. Instructive directives allow for preferences regarding the provision of particular therapies or classes of therapies. *Living wills* are the most common examples of instructive directives, but other types of instructive therapies such as no transfusion and no cardiac pulmonary resuscitation (CPR) directives are also employed. The proxy directive, generally a *Durable Power of Attorney for Health Care*, allows for the designation of a surrogate decision maker of the patient's choosing. This surrogate decision maker makes medical care decisions for the patient in the event he or she is incapacitated (Tonelli et al. 2008).

1. *Power of attorney*
This document gives a person (agent) the authority to authorize a trusted family member or friend to make legal decisions when the principal is no longer competent. There is no standard power of attorney so each one is unique to an individual's situation. The terms of the power of attorney details what authority the caregiver does and does not have. This document should be available for everyone who is affected.

2. *Durable-power-of-attorney for health care*
This document appoints an agent to make all decisions regarding healthcare. These decisions include those regarding providers of healthcare, medical treatment and end-of-life care. This document allows the agent to authorize or refuse any medical treatment for the principal. This power goes into effect once the principal is unable to make decisions for himself or herself and is activated by the principal's attending physician.

3. *Living Will*
A living will allows a person to state what kind of medical care they want to receive. For example, pain relief, comfort care, and what life-support procedures they would like to withhold, for example, resuscitation, foods or fluids. This document is used if a person becomes terminally ill and unable to make his or her wishes known. A terminal illness is defined as one from which a person's physician believes there is no chance of recovery. A living will can also be used if a person becomes permanently unconscious. To be considered permanently unconscious, a person must be viewed as having no reasonable possibility or regaining consciousness or decision-making ability. Two doctors must make this determination. Laws on living wills vary from state to state.

4. *Living Trust*
This document enables a person (called a grantor or trustor) to create a trust and appoint a trustee to carefully invest and manage trust assets once the grantor is no longer able to manage finances. A person can appoint an individual or a financial institution to be a trustee.

5. *Will*
A will is a document created by an individual that names an executor (the person who will manage the estate) and beneficiaries (those who will receive the estate at the time of the person's death).

12.4 Attitudes Toward and Effects of Advance Directives

Advance directives (ADs) have been proposed as a way of facilitating the maintenance of patient autonomy if they become incapacitated in the future. ADs have existed in the U.S. for more than 20 years, yet only 20–30 % of Americans report having an advance directive (Sendensky 2010).[3] And, even when patients have an advance directive physicians are often unaware of their patient's preferences. One large-scale study found that only 25 % of physicians knew that their patients had advance directives on file (Tillyard 2007). A review of the effects that ADs have had on critically ill adults showed little evidence of the effect of ADs on the treatment of acutely ill patients in the intensive care unit. The AD does not facilitate harmonious decision-making at the end of life or maintain an incapacitated patient's autonomy. Physicians therefore frequently consult relatives regarding the appropriateness of treatment interventions, despite data suggesting that the consulted relatives find this emotionally stressful and do not consistently make decisions that accurately reflect their relative's wishes (Tillyard 2007).

A large-scale survey in the U.S. by the Pew Research Center in 2005 found that public awareness of living wills is virtually universal and the number saying that they had a living will more than doubled from 12 % in 1990 to 29 % in 2005

[3] See McIntosh (1999).

(Pew Research Center 2006). People who have helped make end-of-life treatment decisions for loved ones are more likely than others to have a living will or to have discussed their wishes for end-of-life care. And, there is strong sentiment (74 %) in favor of letting close family members decide whether to continue medical treatment for a terminally ill loved one who is unable to communicate their own wishes. Attitudes toward ADs do vary in the U.S. regionally and between states.

A recent cross-sectional survey was conducted in Maryland to determine the prevalence of advance directives (ADs) and identify the enablers and barriers to their adoption. Approximately 34 % of adults in Maryland had an AD. Adults aged 65 and over were more likely to have an AD compared to younger adults (18–64 years). Two times as many Whites than Blacks reported having ADs. Of those who had an AD, the primary motivations for creating one were a personal medical condition or a diagnosis to oneself or a family member/friend. Those without ADs identified their lack of familiarity with them (27 %), being too young or healthy to need one (14 %) or uncertainty about the process for adopting one (11 %) as the major reasons for not having one. Forty percent of the respondents said that they would like to obtain information about ADs from a physician—only 12 % of those who had ADs received the information from their doctors (Pollack et al. 2010).

While these results are from only one state, they point to a need for regulatory and legislative changes to enable more people to learn about ADs. In the U.S., federal law defers to state law about ADs and decision-making, therefore, every state has statutory provisions for ADs (Pollack et al. 2010). As we deal with healthcare reform we need to include advance care planning information so that an informed public can make informed choices about their healthcare goals.[4]

12.5 The Role and Scope of Surrogates in Advance Directives

Sometimes patients are not able to make decisions about their medical care. This applies to newborns, young children, people in transient unconscious states, people in persistent vegetative states, and people with psychiatric or psychological conditions that disrupt ordered thought. Sometimes the incapacity to make decisions is plainly clear to all involved. A patient might be unconscious and is not able to make decisions about surgery, medication, or life support. In those instances the physician is obligated by law to make an inquiry as to whether the patient has executed a power of attorney for healthcare. If there is no person authorized to make medical decisions or that person is unavailable, the physician may turn to surrogate decision makers without a specific court order and without judicial involvement. Physicians may turn to the following persons as surrogate decision-makers as long as they do so in the following order:

[4] See Colello et al. (2009).

- The patient's legal guardian
- The patient's spouse
- Any adult son or daughter
- Either parent
- Any adult brother or sister
- Any adult grandchild
- A close friend
- The guardian of the estate

If multiple decision-makers at the same level are present, for example three adult daughters of the patient, the physician should try to help them reach consensus about a decision. In case of conflict, the majority decision prevails. Treatment decisions for the patient should not be held hostage to families in dispute.

Advance directives come into play only when a patient is unable to communicate his or her wishes. Yet, at the same time surrogate decision-makers must be involved in medical decisions. Surrogate decision-makers can use advance directives as guides when making decisions about a patient. While the advance directive is a guide it comes into play only through a surrogate decision-maker. In some cases surrogate decision-makers may find that the patient's circumstances have changed and is not ethically or legally bound to follow the advance directive as written (Silveira et al. 2010).

In some cases it may not be entirely clear whether someone is able to make medical decisions for themselves or a patient may vary in their mental ability. The point is that some patients lie in a gray area when it comes to their ability to make medical decisions. In these instances physicians may turn to surrogate decision-makers for decisions. In some cases it might be necessary to seek a legal judgment. If courts become involved they use criteria related to formal declarations of competence. Physicians can treat patients without the involvement of a surrogate decision-maker when treatment needs are urgent and no surrogate decision-maker is identified or available (University of Illinois at Chicago School of Medicine 2012).

12.6 Physician Aid-in-Dying

Physicians and family caregivers may care for patients who become so distraught with their immobility, dependency, prognosis, and/or pain that they ask assistance in dying. Physician-aid-in-dying (PAD) refers to a practice in which a physician provides a competent, terminally ill patient with a prescription for a lethal dose of medication, upon a patient's request, which the patient intends to use to end their own life.

Physician-aid-in-dying is not the same as euthanasia or physician-assisted suicide. While both involve the use of lethal medications to deliberately end a patient's life, the major difference is in who acts to end the patient's life. In physician-aid-in-dying, the patient must self-administer the medications; the aid-in-dying refers to a physician providing the medications, but the patient decides whether and when to ingest the lethal medication. Euthanasia is when a third party administers medication or acts directly to end a patient's life. Euthanasia is illegal in all states except Washington (University of Washington School of Medicine 2012).

The ethics of physician-aid-in-dying continues to be debated. Arguments in favor of PAD include: (1) respect for autonomy; (2) justice; (3) compassion; (4) individual liberty vs. state interest; and (5) honesty and transparency. Arguments against PAD include: (1) sanctity of life; (2) passive vs. active distinction; (3) potential for abuse; (4) professional integrity; and (5) fallibility of the profession. Physician-aid-in-dying is legal in Washington and Oregon where voter approved initiatives have legalized aid-in-dying in very specific circumstances.[5]

Legalized physician-aid-in-dying in Oregon is over 10 years old. A 2009 survey of 95 family members of deceased Oregonians who had explicitly requested aid-in-dying showed Oregonians who received a lethal prescription were more likely to believe that their loved one's choices were honored and less likely to have regrets about how their loved one died. Pursuit of aid-in-dying did not appear to have negative effects on surviving members; there was a low prevalence of depression and grief an average of 14 months after the death. This outcome may be associated with greater preparation and acceptance of death (Ganzini et al. 2009).

Tucker (2012), a chest physician, writes that aid-in-dying is increasingly accepted by physicians, and that it is likely more patients will ask about it. She explains that patients approaching death because of a terminal illness may find themselves trapped in a dying process that they find unbearable, even with excellent pain and symptom management. Some patients will want the option of aid-in-dying. The American Medical Women's Association adopted a policy in 2007 in support of aid-in-dying.[6] Tucker provides clinical practice guidelines for physicians responding to patient requests for aid-in-dying.

12.7 Crucial Conversations

Face-to-face conversations between patients and physicians are essential as a patient learns of their terminal condition (Patterson et al. 2002). Conversation is a key component in preserving patients' autonomy and honoring end-of-life wishes. Ideally family caregivers should be present also. A large number of patients and close family members want such a discussion. Yet, there is a seeming ambivalence as to who should initiate the conversation, when, and its focus. Many patients hesitate to

---

[5] Physician aid-in-dying has been legal in Oregon since 1997 and in Washington since 2009. Surveys of individual physicians in practice show that about one in five will receive a request for PAD sometime in their career. Other surveys of physicians show that about half believe that PAD is ethically justified in certain cases. However, professional organizations like the American Medical Association have generally argued against PAD on the grounds that it undermines the integrity of the profession. See http://depts.Washington.edu/bioethx/topics/pad.html. For additional references see Back et al. (1996); Cohen et al. (1994); Ganzini et al. (2000); Ganzini et al. (2001).

[6] See American Medical Women's Association. *American Medical Women's Association Position Paper on Aid in Dying*. http://amwa-doc.org/cms_files/original/Aid_in_Dying1.pdf.

initiate this conversation and so do many physicians.[7] Physicians are trained to maintain health and fight illness and typically have received little guidance on how to communicate about issues surrounding death. Patients and their families sometimes collude to avoid mentioning death or dying even when the patient's suffering is severe and the prognosis is poor (Quill 2000). On the other hand, our society is death-aversive and only reluctantly talks about death as medical failure (Balaban 2000). In some cases it is difficult for patients to even identify "their doctor" let alone the doctor having the time for such a critical discussion. End-of-life discussions should go beyond the narrow focus of resuscitation and address an array of concerns shared by most dying patients and their family caregivers such as fears about dying, end-of-life goals, and attending to physical needs. Good communication can facilitate an end-of-life plan that is medically sound and concordant with the patient's wishes and values. Good communication can help allay fears, minimize pain and experience a peaceful death (Balaban 2000). Specifically, having end-of-life discussions has been found to be associated with higher patient satisfaction with quality of care (Mack et al. 2012). Unfortunately, end-of-life discussions with some patients have occurred about 1 month before death. Earlier end-of-life care discussions could give patients with terminal illnesses a better chance to make decisions about their care (Mack et al. 2012)[8].

Balaban (2000) has suggested a four step approach to guide physicians and family caregivers in a conversation about end-of-life issues. *Step 1* is the physician initiating the discussion with comments to establish a caring connection so that the family and patient feel the physician's empathy and compassion. *Step 2* is clarifying the prognosis, conveying, with directness and compassion, the seriousness of the diagnosis and prognosis, and their limitations. *Step 3* opening the opportunity for the patient to identify their end-of-life goals and special requests for their care. *Step 4* is developing a treatment plan which acknowledges the patient's autonomy, resources, and realities of the progressive condition. One discussion is usually insufficient; patient's preferences are seldom durable over time. Discussing hypothetic scenarios is often useful. The patient and caregiver should feel that the conversation can be continued if needed.

---

[7] See California Healthcare Foundation. Survey results. *Final Chapter: Californians' Attitudes and Experience with Death and Dying*. February 14, 2012. About 80% of Californians said that they would want to discuss end-of-life care with their physicians if they had a serious illness, however, only 7% said they have taken part in such a discussion including 13% of individuals ages 65 and older.

[8] Many cross-cultural differences exist in whether patients and caregivers wish to be fully informed about the patient's diagnosis, prognosis, and treatment options. There are two medical models of care that may influence an individual's beliefs about appropriate communication near the end of life. In the U.S. it was common for physicians not to inform the patient of a poor prognosis or diagnosis. However, the current practice in the U.S. emphasizes full disclosure, self-determination and patient autonomy. Conversely, the model in many Eastern countries emphasizes beneficence and maleficence, with little attention given to patient autonomy. See Moeller et al. (2010).

12.8 Elder Abuse, Neglect and Exploitation in Caregiving

12.8.1 Definition

Sometimes the burden of caregiving becomes overwhelming and results in negative and destructive actions by the caregiver toward the care recipient. Elder mistreatment has been defined as "*Intentional actions that cause harm or create a serious risk of harm, whether or not intended, to a vulnerable elder by a caregiver or other person who stands in a trust relationship to the elder or failure by a caregiver to satisfy the elder's basic needs or to protect the elder from harm*" p. 1 (Bonnie and Wallace 2003). Maltreatment includes physical, sexual, emotional (psychological), or financial abuse, neglect and/or exploitation of a person aged 60 and over.

12.8.2 Prevalence/Incidence of Maltreatment

While elder mistreatment is recognized as a social problem estimates of its scope vary due to an increasing aging and vulnerable population and the methodological difficulties in defining, measuring, and monitoring a complex set of behaviors and situations. The problem is underdiagnosed and underreported. Based on the best estimates between 1 and 2 million Americans age 65 and over have been injured, exploited or otherwise mistreated by someone on whom they depended for their care or protection (Pavlik et al. 2001; Pillemer and Finkelhor 1988). This estimate is similar to others that about 0.5 to 10 % of Americans age 65 and over have experienced mistreatment by a caregiver (Laumann et al. 2008).

The National Elder Abuse Incidence Study (NCEA 1998) based on a representative sample of 20 counties in 15 states reported that:

- Female elders are abused at a higher rate than males, after accounting for their larger proportion in the aging population
- Elders 80 years and older are abused and neglected at two to three times their proportion of the elderly population
- In almost 90 % of the elder abuse and neglect incidents with a known perpetrator, the perpetrator is a family member, and two-thirds of the perpetrators are adult children or spouses
- Victims of self-neglect are usually depressed, confused and/or extremely frail

The National Elder Maltreatment Study was conducted by the National Institute of Justice

(Acierno et al. 2009). The study was a nationally representative sample, based on age, race, and gender, of 5,777 older adults who were interviewed by telephone about a variety of mistreatment types and risk factors. Specific elder mistreatment categories included emotional, physical, sexual, financial, and neglect. It was found that emotional (psychological) mistreatment was the most common event, with one in 20 older adults experiencing this form of abuse in the past year, yet it is rarely reported and emotional maltreatment of elder adults in the workplace may be more common than predicted. Particularly striking was that perpetrators of elder mistreatment were socially isolated and had fewer than three friends. Low income, poor health and low social support all independently predict neglect. Social support emerged as a central protective factor for all forms of elder mistreatment (Leung et al. 2012).

12.8.3 Risk Factors vs. Protective Factors and Elder Maltreatment

Elder maltreatment is not the result of an action or behavior by a perpetrator that recurs without a social context and without factors resulting from the interaction with other people. Precursors or causative factors involve experiences, behaviors, lifestyle or environment, and personal characteristics that increase or decrease the chances that elder maltreatment will occur. Anetzberger (2000) has offered an explanatory model for elder abuse. The model is based on the notion that elder abuse is primarily a function of characteristics of the perpetrator and secondarily characteristics of the victim. Caregiving is the context for the victim-perpetrator interaction, and provides the dynamics that can trigger abuse. Caregiving is not the only context in which elder abuse occurs, however caregiving can provide a fertile ground for victim-perpetrator interactions that may lead to abuse. Elder abuse happens within social interactions that involve a victim-perpetrator dyad. The context of caregiving and the characteristics of the care recipient often provide a care setting of stress and high volatility that can make caregiving particularly difficult (Kohn and Verhoek-Offedahl 2011).

Table 12.1 lists some of the risk factors and protective factors from the published literature on elder maltreatment. In considering the factors and their degree of importance it is necessary to view them not as single or accumulated factors, but their interaction in a given caregiving situation. Caregiving situations vary in recipient characteristics, the environment of caregiving, and how the situation draws out the carer's coping behavior. A stressful caregiving situation may be made less so if a carer has ample and appropriate protective factors to counteract the stress. On the other hand, if the carer has as many problems or issues as the elder they are caring for a stressful situation is likely to be even more stressful. What is key is how and to what degree a carer uses his/her coping skills and resources to turn a possibly volatile and emotive situation into a constructive and helpful one for both the carer and recipient of care.

Caregivers who are stressed can be at risk for engaging in abusive behavior. Stress can come from many sources in addition to caregiving. Regardless of the causes of stress, a stressed caregiver's risk of abusive behavior is high. Anger, coupled with moderate to high levels of depression and resentment increase the risk of abusive behavior significantly (McNeil et al. 2010).

Abusive behavior has been linked to the degree of cognitive impairment of the care recipient. Having fewer symptoms of dementia has been found to be protective for verbal abuse. As dementia progresses the recipient is at increased risk of being

Table 12.1 Risk factors and protective factors for elder maltreatment. (Source: Adapted from Campbell Reay and Browne 2001)

Risk factors	Protective factors
Responsible for elderly dependent aged 75 or older	Carer takes respite
Carer lives with elderly dependent	Carer has good family support and friends
Inexperienced or unwilling caregiver	Carer has spiritual beliefs and practices
Carer who has high expectations of the elderly dependent	Carer has nutritional diet, adequate physical exercise, restful sleep
Carer who has other caregiving demands, e.g. spouse or children	Carer has hobbies, relaxation, meditation time
Carer who is isolated and has minimal or no family support; negative family relationships	Carer has community resources to draw on
Carer who has poor physical health	Carer has sources of advice, assistance
Carer who has a history of depression	Carer has good self-control
Carer who has a history of anxiety	Carer is optimistic, hopeful
Carer who has a history of alcohol abuse	
Carer who has a history of drug abuse	
Carer who was abused/neglected as a child or where there was a history of family violence	
Carer who is subject to high stress and strain	
Carer who has a relationship conflict	
Carer who is impulsive/impatient	
Carer with high degree of resentment/anger	

verbally abused. Verbally abusive behavior on the part of the carer has been found to be related to verbally abusive behavior by the care recipient (Vande Weerd and Paveza 2005). Interestingly, abusive behavior toward elderly people with dementia is not considered by abusers to be as serious as that toward elderly people without dementia (Matsuda 2007). Maintaining safety and respect for human rights is sometimes difficult in the care of persons with dementia, although no level of violence is acceptable. Matsuda (2007) suggests that efforts to abolish the prejudice against dementia is necessary if we are to reduce the risk of abuse. Bonnie and Wallace (2003) suggest that dementia itself is not a risk factor for carer abuse, but rather the disruptive behaviors that result from dementia. This is consistent with research that has shown disruptive behaviors by Alzheimer's patients to be an especially strong cause of caregiver stress.

12.9 Elder Maltreatment in Institutional Settings

Despite the likelihood that elder maltreatment in institutional settings is equally or more prevalent than abuse in domestic settings only one study has been conducted that specifically addressed risk factors. Pillemer and Bachman-Prehn (1991) examined data from a survey of staff regarding self-reported psychological and physical abuse (Bonnie and Wallace 2003; Gorbien and Einsenstein 2005). Predictors of psychological abuse were staff burnout, experiencing aggression from residents, negative attitudes toward residents, and age of the staff member, with younger staff more likely to engage in psychological abuse. Risk factors for physical abuse were also staff burnout and resident aggression. This study is limited by the self-report method and resulting bias since staff would have to report themselves or their fellow caregivers. Determining the true incidence and prevalence of elder abuse is difficult due to underreporting, varying definitions, and the lack of uniform processes among reporting agencies. In addition, various states have different reporting methods and requirements. The United States General Accounting Office (GAO) (2002) reported that allegations of abuse are not reported promptly, local law enforcement officials are seldom summoned to nursing homes to investigate allegations of abuse, and few allegations are prosecuted.[9]

The characteristics of residents of long-term care facilities put them at risk for maltreatment. Vulnerability results from dependency on caregivers due to chronic medical illnesses, especially those that affect cognition (Gibbs and Mosqueda 2004). A 1999 national survey of nursing homes revealed that 32 % of residents in nursing facilities required assistance with four activities of daily living (ADLs), and 75 % required assistance with at least three ADLs (Jones 2002). Studies continue to provide evidence that persons with dementia carry a high risk for maltreatment. Persons with behavioral problems are also at high risk.

Studies of abusive caregivers in long-term care facilities have been largely based on surveys. Perpetrators of abuse may not perceive certain behaviors as abusive. Many abusers believe that combative behavior by residents is intentional and that responses by staff were justified as self-defense and not considered abusive (Gibbs and Mosqueda 2004).

Other factors strongly associated with abusive behavior include an unwilling or inexperienced caregiver, a relationship conflict, high strain, isolation, substance abuse, mental illness, and a history of transgenerational violence. Employment background checks do not provide adequate protection against maltreatment. Some states require a criminal background check, others do not. But frequently such checks do not uncover convictions in another state (Gibbs and Mosqueda 2004).

Neglect is more difficult to detect compared to other types of abuse as the signs of neglect are often mistakenly attributed to aging or the complications of illness. Markers for neglect include pressure ulcers, malnutrition, dehydration, failure to treat pain and withholding feeding assistance. Passive neglect may occur if caregivers do not recognize a potentially life-threatening situation. Severely impaired persons have difficulty communicating; subtle changes in appetite, alertness and personality can be important signs of end-stage disease and the need for comfort care (Gibbs and Mosqueda 2004).

Many experts agree that ways to help reduce elder abuse and neglect are to increase nursing ratios, increase staff training, improve supervisory oversight, enhance screening and hiring practices, and monitor stress factors in the working environment.

---

[9] The National Center on Elder Abuse (NCEA) serves as a national resource center dedicated to the prevention of elder mistreatment. http://www.aoa.gov/AoA_programs/Elder_Rights/NCEA/index.aspx.

12.10 Summary

Ethical and legal issues are embedded in the role of family caregiver. Caregiving is a commitment to maintain the care and well-being of a loved one for an indeterminate period of time, often resulting in changes in the recipient's total care until death. As the key decision-maker the family caregiver is faced with choosing options in addressing the concerns and expectations of the recipient and/or other family members, and their own limitations in skills, time and resources. Decision-making and planning for incapacity, long-term care, and death usually do not occur in advance of an event, therefore, it is not surprising that only 20–30 % of Americans have formalized their wishes in the event of their incapacity or death.

Decision-making about the future usually occurs at the time of a diagnosis of a terminal illness. Physicians honor the principle of patient autonomy about decisions affecting their lives. A conversation about advance directives and questions about caregiving should involve the physician, patient, and family caregiver. The openness and frankness of this conversation can prevent future misunderstanding as the needs for care increase. Preparing power of attorney, durable power of attorney for healthcare, and living will and living trust papers is important and should be carried out as soon as possible. Advance directives help to preserve the recipient's well-being by protecting them from unwanted medical interventions, and allow the caregiver to pursue recipient's wishes.

Advance directives come into play only when the care recipient is unable to communicate their wishes. Yet, surrogate decision-makers must be involved in medical decisions. Physicians can treat patients without the involvement of a surrogate decision-maker when treatment needs are urgent and no surrogate decision-maker is identified or available.

In the process of caregiving the recipient may become so distraught with their pain, prognosis, and dependency that they ask for assistance in dying from their physician. Physician-aid-in-dying is illegal in all states except Washington and Oregon where voters approved initiatives that have legalized aid-in-dying in very specific circumstances. This is why face-to-face conversations between patients and physicians are important as soon as a person learns of their terminal condition. Conversation is critical in preserving the person's autonomy, clarifying his/her expectations, and end-of-life wishes.

Sometimes the burden of caregiving becomes overwhelming and results in negative and destructive behavior by the caregiver. Elder maltreatment includes physical, psychological, sexual, or financial abuse, neglect and/or exploitation of a person aged 60 and over. The problem is underdiagnosed and underreported, but estimates range from 0.5–10 % of Americans 65 and over who are thought to have experienced maltreatment.

Caregivers who are stressed can be at risk for engaging in abusive behavior. Abusive behavior has been linked to the degree of cognitive impairment of the care recipient. Verbally abusive behavior by the carer has been found to be related to verbal abuse by the care recipient. Interestingly, abusive behavior toward the elderly with dementia is not considered by abusers to be as serious as that toward elderly people without dementia. Female elders are abused at a higher rate than males. Elders 80 years and older are abused and neglected at two to three times their proportion of the elderly population. In almost 90 % of the known cases of elder abuse and neglect the perpetrator is a family member. Victims of self-neglect are usually depressed, confused, and/or extremely frail. The National Elder Maltreatment Study in 2009 found that emotional maltreatment was the most common event, with one in 20 older adults experiencing this form of abuse.

Elder maltreatment is considered to be as equally, or more, prevalent in institutional settings. Risk factors for physical abuse include staff burnout, resident aggression, and the age of the carer, with younger staff more likely to engage in emotional or psychological abuse. The characteristics of residents of long-term care facilities put them at risk for maltreatment. Neglect is more difficult to detect compared to other types of abuse because the signs of neglect are more readily attributed to aging or the complications of disease.

Many experts agree that ways to prevent abuse and neglect are to increase staffing ratios, more staff training, increasing supervisory oversight, improve screening and hiring practices, and monitor stress in the working environment.

12.11 Questions for Discussion

1. What are some ways to increase the number of people who have Advance Directives? Discuss barriers and how to overcome them.
2. Why are some physicians reluctant to refer to hospice? Discuss.
3. Discuss the major ethical and legal issues surrounding physician aid-in-dying.
4. What are the caregiver risks for elder maltreatment?
5. Discuss interventions to reduce the risks for elder maltreatment.

References

Acierno, R., Hernandez-Tejada, M., Muzzy, W., & Steve, K. (2009). *The national elder maltreatment study final report* Document No. 226456. National Institute of Justice. Washington, DC. http://www.ncjrs.gov/pdffiles1/nig/grants/226456.pdf. Accessed 25 August 2012.

Anetzberger, G. J. (2000). Caregiving: Primary cause of elder abuse? *Generations, Summer,* 46–51.

Back, A. L., et al. (1996). Physician-assisted suicide and euthanasia in Washington State. Patient requests and physician responses. *Journal of the American Medical Association, 275*(12), 919–925.

Balaban, R. B. (2000). A physician's guide to talking about end-of-life care. *Journal of General Internal Medicine, 15*(3), 195–200.

Bonnie, R. J., & Wallace, R. B. (Eds.). (2003). *Elder mistreatment: Abuse, neglect, and exploitation in an aging America.* (Committee on National Statistics and Committee on Law and Justice, Division of Behavioral and Social Sciences and Education. National Research Council). Washington, DC: The National Academies Press.

Buchanan, A. E., & Brock, D. W. (1989). *Deciding for others: The ethics of surrogate decision-making.* New York: Cambridge University Press.

Campbell Reay, A. M., & Browne, K. D. (2001). Risk factor characteristics in carers who physically abuse or neglect their elderly dependents. *Aging & Mental Health, 5*(1), 56–62.
Cohen, J. S., et al. (1994). Attitudes toward assisted suicide and euthanasia among physicians in Washington state. *New England Journal of Medicine, 331*(2), 89–94.
Colello, K. J., Mulvey, J., Sarata, A. K., Williams, E. D., & Thomas, K. R. (2009). End-of-life care; Services, costs, ethics, and quality of care. Congressional Research Service. Report 7-5700: February 23, 2009.
Ganzini, L., et al. (2000). Physicians' experiences with the Oregon Death with Dignity Act. *New England Journal of Medicine, 342*(8), 557–563.
Ganzini, L., et al. (2001). Oregon physicians' attitudes about and experiences with end-of-life care since passage of the Oregon Death with Dignity Act. *Journal of the American Medical Association, 285*(18), 2363–2369.
Ganzini, L., Goy, E. R., Dobscha, S. K., & Prigerson, H. (2009). Mental health outcomes of family members of Oregonians who request physician aid in dying. *Journal of Pain and Symptom Management, 38*(6), 807–815.
Gessert, C. E. (2008). The problem with autonomy: An overemphasis on patient autonomy results in patients feeling abandoned and physicians feeling frustrated. Minnesota medicine, April. http://www.minnesotamedicine.com/Pastissues2008/April2008/CommentaryApril2008.aspx. Accessed 5 August 2012.
Gibbs, L. M., & Mosqueda, L. (2004). Confronting elder maltreatment in long-term care. *Annals of Long-Term Care, 12*(4), 30–35.
Gorbien, M. J., & Einsenstein, A. R. (2005). Elder abuse and neglect: An overview. *Clinics in Geriatric Medicine, 21*(2), 279–292.
Hebert, L. E., Scherr, P. A., Beckett, L. A., et al. (1995). Age-specific incidence of Alzheimer's disease in a community population. *Journals of the American Medical Association, 273*(17), 1354–1359.
Jones, A. (2002). The national nursing home survey: 1999 summary, National Center of Health Statistics. *Vital Health Statistics, 13*(152), 1–116.
Kapp, M. B. (1991). Legal and ethical issues in family caregiving and the role of public policy. *Home Health Care Services Quarterly, 12*(4), 5–28.
Kohn, R., & Verhoek-Oftedahl, W. (2011). Caregiving and elder abuse. *Medicine & Health/Rhode Island, 94*(2), 47–49.
Kuczewski, M. G., & Polansky, R. (Eds.). (2000). *Bioethics: Ancient themes in contemporary issues.* Cambridge: MIT Press.
Laumann, E. O., Leitsch, S. A., & Waite, L. J. (2008). Elder mistreatment in the United States: Prevalence estimates from a nationally representative study. *Journal of Gerontology, 638*(4), S248–254.
Leung, J. M., Udris, E. M., Uman, J., & Au, D. H. (2012). The effect of end-of-life discussions on perceived quality of care and health status among patients with COPD. *Chest, 142*(1), 128–133.
Mack, J. W., Weeks, J. C., Wright, A. A., et al. (2010). End-of-life discussions, goal attainment, and distress at the end-of-life: Predictors and outcomes of receipt of care consistent with preferences. *Journal of Clinical Oncology, 28*(7), 1203–1208.
Mack, J. W., Cronin, A., Taback, N., et al. (2012). End-of-life care discussions among patients with advanced cancer: A cohort study. *Annals of Internal Medicine, 156,* 204–210.
Matsuda, O. (2007). An assessment of the attitudes of potential caregivers toward the abuse of elderly persons with and without dementia. *Int Psychogeriatr, 19*(5): 892-901.
McIntosh, J. L. (1999). Death and dying across the life span. In T. L. Whitman, T. V. Merluzzi, & R. D. White (Eds.), *Life-span perspectives on health and illness* (pp. 249–274). Mahwah: Lawrence Erlbaum Associates.
McNeil, G., Kosberg, J., Durkin, D. W., Deroster, J., & Williamson, G. M. (2010). Caregiver mental health and potentially harmful caregiving behavior: The central role of caregiver anger. *The Gerontologist, 50*(1), 76–86.
Moeller, J. R., Lewis, M. M., & Werth, J. L. (2010). End-of-life issues. In J. C. Cavanaugh & C. K. Cavanaugh (Eds.), *Aging in America, Vol. 1 Psychological aspects.* Santa Barbara: ABC–CLIO.

National Center on Elder Abuse (NCEA). (1998). National Center on Elder Abuse (NCEA) at The American Public Health Human Services Association in collaboration with Westat, Inc. Final Report, September, 1998. http://www.aoa.gov/AoARoot/AoA_Programe/Elder_Rights/Elder_Abuse/docs/ABuseReport_Full.pdf. Accessed 25 August 2012.

Patterson, K., Grenny, J., McMillan, R., & Switzler, A. (2002). *Crucial conversations: Tools for talking when stakes are high.* New York: McGraw Hill.

Pavlik, V. N., Hyman, D. J., Festa, N. A., & Dyer, C. B. (2001). Quantifying the problem of abuse and neglect in adults-analysis of a state wide database. *Journal of the American Geriatrics Society, 49*(1), 45–48.

Pew Research Center. (2006). Strong public support for right to die. Summary of findings. January 6, 2006. http://www.people-press.org/2006/01/05/strong-public-support-for-right-to-die/. Accessed 13 August 2012.

Pillemer, K., & Bachman-Prehn, R. (1991). Helping and hurting: Predictors of maltreatment of patients in nursing homes. *Research on Aging, 13,* 74–95.

Pillemer, K. A., & Finkelhor, D. (1988). The prevalence of elder abuse: A random sample survey. *The Gerontologist, 28*(1), 51–57.

Pollack, K. M., Morhaim, D., & Williams, M. A. (2010). The public's perspectives on advance directives: Implications for state legislative and regulatory policy. *Health Policy (Amsterdam, Netherlands), 96,* 57–63.

Quill, T. E. (2000). Initiating end-of-life discussions with seriously ill patients. Addressing the "elephant in the room." *Journal of the American Medical Association, 284*(19), 2502–2507.

Sendensky, M. (2010). 5 years after Schiavo, few make end-of-life plans. Boston.com. Accessed 10 March 2010.

Silveira, M. J., Kim, S. Y. H., & Langa, K. M. (2010). Advance directives and outcomes of surrogate decision-making before death. *New England Journal of Medicine, 362*(13), 1211–1218.

Tillyard, A. R. J. (2007). Ethics review: 'Living wills' and intensive care-an overview of the American experience. *Critical Care, 11,* 219.

Tonelli, M. K., Braddock, C. H., & Edwards, K. A. (2008). Advance directives. http://depts.washington.edu/bioethx/topics/advdir.htm. Accessed 15 August 2012.

Tucker, K. L. (2012). Aid in dying: Guidance for an emerging end-of-life practice. *Chest, 142*(1), 218–224.

U.S. Government Accounting Office (GAO). (2002). *Nursing homes: More can be done to protect residents from abuse.* GAO-02-448T, March, 1, 2002.

University of Illinois College of Medicine. (2012). http://www.uic.edu/depts/mcam/ethics/surrogate.htm. Accessed 18 August 2012.

University of Washington School of Medicine. (2012). http://depts.washington.edu/bioethx/topics/pad.html. Accessed 20 August 2012.

Vande Weerd, C., & Paveza, G. J. (2005). Verbal mistreatment in older adults: A look at persons with Alzheimer's disease and their caregivers in the state of Florida. *Journal of Elder Abuse & Neglect, 17*(4), 1–30.

Winzelberg, G. S., Hanson, L. C., & Tulsky, J. A. (2005). Beyond autonomy: Diversifying end-of-life decision-making approaches to serve patients and families. *Journal of the American Geriatrics Society, 53*(6), 1046–1050.

Chapter 13
National Caregiving Policy Initiatives

13.1 Introduction

Both the numbers of older people and their proportion of the total U.S. population are increasing and will continue to do so for decades to come. While there is widespread agreement that these increasing numbers give greater importance to policy decisions that affect the elderly, especially decisions regarding entitlements, this is where agreement stops. Policymakers disagree about the obligations of government and the responsibilities of individuals, about the contributions of older people and their expectations and demands for receiving long-term healthcare (Rowe and Kahn 1998; Rowe 2011; Hudson 2011). We too often learn how to protect our health after it is compromised and when affordability and coverage of health services are limited (McGlynn et al. 2008).[1] Even those persons who age successfully encounter general health decline in old age which requires some degree of informal caregiving services. Family caregivers are the principal providers of such services and are key players in coordinating healthcare for family members (O'Shaughnessy 2012).

Historically, as a society, we have relied on home-based healthcare with family members and other informal providers being the principal caregivers and coordinators of health and social services. However, this arrangement is no longer an effective or efficient method of providing assistance to people with functional limitations and chronic impairments (O'Shaughnessy 2012). Long-term care has become an increasingly urgent policy issue (Elmore and Talley 2009; Mechanic 2006; Stone 2000; Feinberg et al. 2011). The objective is not to minimize the importance of the home and family members in care but rather to support them as partners in a coordinated system of care involving professional caregivers and community-based resources.

Americans who provide care for aging parents lose an estimated 3 trillion $ in wages, pension, and Social Security benefits when they take time off to do so. Nearly 10 million adult children over the age of 50 care for their aging parents. As the demand for caregivers increases there will be a need for employers and policymakers

[1] See the interesting article on how society shapes aging by Berkman and Glymour (2006). Also see Mechanic (2006, pp. 51–66).

J. G. Bruhn, H. M. Rebach, *The Sociology of Caregiving*,
Clinical Sociology: Research and Practice, DOI 10.1007/978-94-017-8857-1_13,

to accommodate the needs of working caregivers (Metlife Mature Market Institute 2008). It seems that it is not the irresolvable gaps in our knowledge or administrative capacities, but rather political and ideological disagreement about the proper direction of change that is inhibiting the formulation of a national healthcare policy that comprehensively addresses the caregiving needs of the aging in our society (Hacker 2008).

The objectives of this chapter are to: (1) suggest principles that should drive a comprehensive national caregiving policy; (2) present current federal and state initiatives for caregiving; and (3) offer recommendations for improving caregiving services to an aging population based on common features of innovative models which have been successful.

13.1.1 Caregiving Principles and National Health Policy

Family caregiving continues to be an essential part of the care of aging and disabled persons in our society. However, demographic and social changes have created new demands on family caregivers which affect their availability, accessibility and affordability so that they are less able to take on the role of family caregiver. In addition, the increased longevity of family members with complex chronic conditions has extended the role of family caregivers to the degree that this responsibility impinges on the caregiver's own health and longevity. There is a need for a national healthcare policy that addresses the needs of an aging society with a shortage of caregivers (Mintz et al. 2003).

Some general principles governing caregiving have been proposed. In December, 2003, Suzanne Mintz assembled a collaborative group of family caregiver advocates who developed eight principles of public policy that should underlie caregiving in all situations.[2] These principles, while broadly applicable, would be implemented as appropriate to various caregiving settings (Mintz et al. 2003).

Principle 1

Family caregiving concerns must be a central component of healthcare, long-term care, and social service policymaking. Family caregivers are the most neglected group of the health and long-term care system. In return for family caregivers' contributions to the public good, society, through its public and private sectors, must support caregivers through well-designed policies, programs, and practice.

Principle 2

Family caregivers must be protected against the financial, physical, and emotional consequences of caregiving that can put their own health and well-being in

---

[2] The group was comprised of Lynn Friss Feinberg of the National Center on Caregiving/Family Caregiving Alliance; Jane Horvath, a health policy analyst; Gail Hunt and Les Plooster of the National Alliance for Caregiving; Jill Kagan of the National Respite Coalition; Carol Levine of the Families and Healthcare Project, United Fund; Joanne Lynn MD of Americans for Better Care of the Dying; Suzanne Mintz of the National Family Caregivers Association; and Ann Wilkinson of the Rand Corporation.

jeopardy. There is substantial evidence that family caregivers serve in their role at significant physical, psychological and financial losses due to the stress of their job as a caregiver (see Chap. 11 The Health of Caregivers in this text).

Principle 3

Family caregivers must have access to affordable, readily available, high quality respite care as a key component of the supportive services network. Respite is not always accessible to the family because of eligibility requirements, geographic barriers, cost, or the lack of culturally sensitive programs. Therefore, systems need to be in place to identify and coordinate federal, state and community-based respite resources for the family.

Principle 4

Family caregivers must be supported by family-friendly policies in the workplace such as flextime, work-at-home options, job sharing, employer paid services, etc. Family caregivers are doubly penalized and may have to leave the workforce for caregiving.

Principle 5

Family caregivers must have appropriate, timely, and ongoing education and training in order to successfully meet their caregiving responsibilities and to be advocates for their loved ones across care settings. Family caregivers' need for information and training changes throughout the course of their loved one's illness. They must have opportunities to learn new skills as they become necessary, access new resources and learn about options for care as the situation changes. Families need honest information in understandable, nonjudgmental and culturally sensitive ways.

Principle 6

Family caregivers and their loved ones must have affordable, readily available, high quality, comprehensive services that are coordinated across all care settings. There is a need for coordination of information and services within each system and between systems of care. Many people require services from many parts of the medical and long-term care systems. Sometimes conflicting and confusing information is given resulting in poor care coordination leading to unnecessary treatment or other intervention.

Principle 7

Family caregivers and their loved ones must be assured of an affordable, well-qualified, and sustainable healthcare workforce across all care settings. A shortage of well qualified, reliable, and affordable healthcare workers has a direct effect on the health and safety of persons with chronic conditions or disabilities and on the health and well-being of family caregivers.

Principle 8

Family caregivers must have access to regular comprehensive assessments of their caregiving to determine what assistance they may require. Family caregiving should be considered an integral part of the long-term care system, as individuals with rights to their own support and assessments of their needs. The availability of family members or others to provide uncompensated care should not be considered in allocating long-term care benefits as in the Medicaid program.

The past decade has witnessed an increase in both policy initiatives to enhance support services for family caregivers and in professional recognition of family caregivers as partners in care. Although some observers contend that families are on their own to a greater degree today than in the past, caregiving is now embedded in several key initiatives at the federal and state levels (Feinberg et al. 2011; Kelly 2010).

13.2 National Initiatives in Caregiving

13.2.1 The National Family Caregiver Support Program (NFCSP) (2000) Under the Older Americans Act Title ITTE

The eight principles of public policy were developed about the same time as a federal initiative, The National Family Caregiver Support Program (NFCSP), was established in 2000 under the U.S. Administration on Aging, with an initial budget in 2001 of $ 155.2 million. The NFCSP provides grants to States and territories, based on their share of the population aged 60 and over, to fund a range of supports that assist families and informal caregivers including grandparents and older relatives who raise children,[3] to care for their loved ones at home for as long as possible. Under this program States can provide the following services:

- Information to caregivers about available services
- Assistance to caregivers in gaining access to services
- Individual counseling, organization of support groups, and caregiver training
- Respite care
- Supplemental services on a limited basis.

These services work in conjunction with other State and community-based services to provide a coordinated system of supports. Studies have shown that these services can reduce caregiver depression, anxiety and stress and enable them to provide care longer, thereby avoiding or delaying the need for costly institutional care.

From 2001–2003, following the initial funding of NFCSP, Feinberg and Newman (2004) selected 10 States as case studies to develop an extensive survey to profile federal and state programs in the 50 States and District of Columbia. Conclusions from the 50 State Study were that there was an increasing availability of publically funded caregiver support services and options for family caregivers across the States and within States. The NFCSP was emerging as a key program to enhance the scope of caregiver support services and is fueling innovation in the States, but was inadequately funded ($ 138.7 M in 2003). While there was great

[3] See *A Guide to the National Family Support Program and its Inclusion of Grandparents and Other Relatives Raising Children*. 2nd edition, September, 2003. Generations United, Washington, DC. guogu.org.

variation among States and programs within States, there was a broad recognition of the value of uniformly assessing caregiver needs and the importance of training and technical assistance in this area. States have mixed views on approaches to systems development and the importance of caregiver support services within home and community-based care, and integrating family caregiving programs into home and community-based programs. Feinberg et al. (2004) concluded that future next steps include: (1) increase funding to reduce gaps in support services; (2) improve data collection and reporting; (3) strengthen and expand the uniform assessment of caregiver needs in all NFCSP programs; (4) conduct a national public awareness campaign on family caregiving; and (5) invest in innovation, promising practices, and technical assistance.

13.2.2 The Affordable Care Act of 2010 (P.L. 111–148)

On March 23, 2010 President Obama signed comprehensive health reform, the Patient Protection and Affordable Care Act, into law. A summary of the law, and changes made to the law by subsequent legislation, focuses on provisions to expand coverage, control healthcare costs, and improve the healthcare delivery system can be found elsewhere (Kaiser Family Foundation 2010). The features of the law discussed here are those that bear most on caregiving (Table 13.1).

This new healthcare law promotes the central importance of person and family-centered care in the design and delivery of new models of care to improve the quality and efficiency of healthcare, including the assessment of the family caregiver's experience of care.[4]

a. *Building a Long-Term Care Workforce*

The Affordable Care Act establishes six initiatives towards building a long-term care workforce.

1. Establishes a system for comprehensive healthcare planning which will advise Congress on healthcare workforce needs and policies that are needed to address those needs. This will help policy makers to develop strategies to address workforce shortages such as long-term care workers.
2. Establishes a National Center for Healthcare Workforce Analysis which will develop the workforce supply and demand data that are needed to create a comprehensive workforce strategy.
3. Establishes a program to provide grants to States to develop and carry out workforce planning, including planning for a long-term care workforce.

[4] The Affordable Care Act also provides the opportunity to redesign the nation's mental health system. It promotes new programs such as health homes, interdisciplinary care teams, the co-location of physical health and behavioral services, collaborative care, and the broadening of the Medicaid Home and Community-based Services option. The Act offers the opportunity to insure more people, reimburse previously unreimbursed services, integrate care, confront complex chronic comorbidities, and adopt underused evidence-based interventions (See Mechanic 2012).

Table 13.1 Understanding the Patient Protection and Affordable Care Act of 2010. (Source: National Physicians Alliance Foundation www.npafoundation.org. Accessed 22 Jan 2013)

Provisions that began in 2010
Coverage for kids with pre-existing conditions, and new options for young adults
Insurance companies can no longer deny coverage to children due to a pre-existing condition like asthma or diabetes. Young adults can now stay on their parent's insurance plan up to age 26, regardless of whether that young adult is married
No more lifetime caps and annual limits
Insurance companies can no longer set lifetime limits or unreasonable annual limits on the dollar value of benefits. This is important for Americans with health conditions that require expensive medications and treatments. Lifetime caps are now prohibited effective 2010. All annual limits will be completely banned by 2014
Keeping your coverage when you get sick
Thousands of people with health insurance have fallen ill only to find that their insurance companies suddenly cancel their coverage. This process, where an insurance company drops an enrollee, also called rescission, is now prohibited
Better prescription drug coverage for seniors
In 2010, more than 1 million seniors received $ 250 checks to help pay for their Medicare prescription drug coverage. The checks were paid to seniors who fell into the coverage gap known as the "doughnut hole." The doughnut hole will be eliminated by 2020 (see 2011 for more about improved drug coverage for seniors)
New option for adults with costly medical needs
Until 2014, adults who are refused an insurance policy because of a pre-existing condition can purchase subsidized health insurance from a new nationwide high-risk pool. Participating insurance plans must pay at least 65 % of medical costs. Starting in 2014, insurance companies will no longer be allowed to refuse coverage for adults due to a pre-existing condition
Tax credits for small businesses
Health Insurance tax credits are now available for businesses with 25 or fewer employees and with average wages below $ 50,000. The credit will cover up to 35 % of the employer's contribution to employee health benefits. In 2014, the credit will cover up to 50 % of premium costs for participating employers
No-cost preventive care
Preventive care, like immunizations, blood tests and mammograms, is now free of charge. Medicare and private health insurance plans can no longer require cost-sharing, like co-pays, for preventive care. By improving access to preventive services, doctors can treat their patients' healthcare needs at earlier stages and better prevent dangerous consequences
Retiree health benefits
Employers can apply for subsidies to help cover the cost of retiree health benefits, until retirees are eligible for Medicare. The subsidies can cover up to 80 % of retiree costs
Regulating premium increases
Federal and state governments are now reviewing annual premium increases. Insurance companies are required to justify premium increases to regulators, and to post this information on the web. Insurance companies with unfair premium increases may be excluded from participating in the state insurance exchanges, a form of "one-stop shopping" for insurance that begins in 2014. The exchanges will offer new insurance options for families and small businesses
Requiring insurance companies to spend your premium payments on medical care
Insurance companies must now meet new efficiency standards, saving you money. Starting in 2011, if insurance companies spend more than 15 to 20 % of your premium payments on non-medical costs, like administration, they must offer you a rebate
Federal Medicaid help for states and low income families
States are now approved to provide Medicaid coverage to adults with or without children up to 133 % of the federal poverty level. States that do so will receive current federal matching rates to cover additional costs. Medicaid is a joint federal-state healthcare program

Table 13.1 (continued)

Provisions that began in 2010
2011 and beyond
Better and fairer insurance coverage for all Americans
Starting in 2014, insurance companies cannot deny coverage to anyone based on pre-existing medical conditions. They cannot consider your health status when setting the price of your premiums. The maximum time a person will have to wait for their coverage to take effect will be 90 days. And, new regulations will require insurance companies to more fairly distribute costs so that people trying to buy insurance are not "priced out" of the market
Health insurance tax subsidies for families
In 2014, middle income individuals and families earning less than 400 % of the federal poverty level will receive subsidies to help them purchase health insurance. These subsidies will lower the cost of premiums. Out-of-pocket expenses will also be reduced for these individuals and families
Improving the Medicare Rx drug program
Medicare enrollees in the "doughnut hole" can get 50 % discounts on all brand-name drugs in 2011. The "doughnut hole"—the gap in coverage in Medicare's prescription drug program—will be eliminated by 2020
Less insurance company paperwork
Starting in 2013, insurance companies must use simpler and standardized paperwork. Reducing and eliminating complex paperwork will improve efficiency and communications between healthcare organizations, doctors, and insurance companies
Purchasing health insurance across state lines
In 2016, two or more states can allow qualifying health insurance plans to be purchased across state lines.
New options for insurance—state health insurance exchanges
Starting in 2014, states will launch new health insurance "exchanges" for individuals and small businesses to purchase health insurance. Insurance offered in these "exchanges" will meet standards for benefits, quality, and reliability. Consumers will be able to keep their existing insurance, or purchase new coverage options in the "exchange"

4. Provides new grants to encourage people to train to be long-term care workers. Grant recipients need to make a minimum 2 year service commitment.
5. Establishes a voluntary long-term care insurance program and requires States to provide the infrastructure to support the development of a larger personal attendant workforce to meet the needs of an aging population.
6. Establishes a grant program for long-term care facilities to develop training, career advancement, and staff retention programs. This includes funding for demonstration projects to determine the best ways to improve training and retention among these workers.

b. *A New Voluntary Long-Term Care Insurance Program*

This part of the Affordable Care Act establishes the first federal, voluntary long-term care insurance program for working adults that will provide a cash benefit to enrollees who have been in the program for at least 5 years and who need long-term care services. It will be fully funded by enrollee premiums.

c. *Programs that Give States Incentives to Expand Home and Community-Based Services in Medicaid*

1. The Affordable Care Act creates a new optional program called the State Balancing Initiative Payments Program, open to States that spend less than 50% of their Medicaid long-term services dollars on non-institutional care. It provides an added Medicaid match for States to develop administrative programs that have been shown to increase the use of home- and community-based services in Medicaid.
2. The Affordable Care Act creates a new optional program called the Community First Choice Option. This is a new program that States can add to their Medicaid programs. It allows States to offer a broad range of personal attendant services to Medicaid beneficiaries who are living in the community. It also covers supports such as assistance devices and training, if their use would reduce the need for personal attendants. It is designed to help more people in Medicaid to continue living in their homes or in the community, rather than having to move to a nursing facility.

d. *Programs to Improve Resources that Help Caregivers and Consumers*

1. The Affordable Care Act provides additional funding for States to expand their aging and disability resource centers. These centers provide information on care options, help people connect with services, and give advice on options to finance care.
2. The Affordable Care Act requires improvements to the Nursing Home Compare Website. The new law outlines information that nursing homes must provide, including information on staffing levels, complaints filed against the facility, adjudications, and outcomes; and plans for corrective action.

e. *Programs that Protect Seniors and People with Disabilities*

1. The Affordable Care Act provides new funding for State adult protective services offices to develop national strategies to combat elder abuse, to enhance the services that are provided by adult protective services offices, and to fund demonstration projects that test new methods to track elder abuse, neglect and financial exploitation. Funding is also available for State long-term care ombudsman offices to conduct training programs on abuse detection.
2. The Department of Health and Human Services will establish a national criminal background check program for prospective long-term care employees who apply to work directly with patients. This is expected to improve patient care and reduce abuse.

f. *Programs that Improve Nursing Home Care*

1. Nursing facilities must now conduct dementia management and abuse prevention training for all new employees. The Secretary of Health and Human Services has the option of requiring facilities to conduct ongoing training.
2. Until the passage of the Affordable Care Act there was no requirement that nursing facilities have compliance or ethics programs for staff. Facilities must develop programs to train staff regarding care standards and identifying and reporting abuse.

3. The Affordable Care Act provides funds for demonstration projects to test different nursing home care models. The results should help improve nursing home care.
4. Nursing facilities have closed without making adequate provisions for the ongoing care of residents. Nursing facilities are now required to provide at least 60 days' notice of closure to the State long-term care ombudsman office, the Secretary of Health and Human Services, and residents and their representatives. The notice must include plans for relocating residents. If needed, Medicare and Medicaid payments to nursing homes may continue while patients are relocated.
5. The Affordable Care Act establishes a pilot program to oversee nursing facility chains that operate in several States. The Office of the Inspector General and the Department of Health and Human Services will work together to develop and operate this program (Families USA 2011; Feinberg et al. 2011; O'Shaughnessy 2012).

13.2.3 Caregivers and Veteran Omnibus Health Services Act of 2010 (P.L. 111–163)

In 2010 President Obama signed the above Act into law. This new law authorizes several initiatives related to service members, veterans, and their families, with a particular focus on caregivers of veterans, mental health services, women veterans, homeless veterans, veterans in rural areas, and research and education. The law authorizes the following related to caregivers of veterans:

- Training in providing personal care service to the veteran
- Ongoing technical support
- Counseling
- Lodging when accompanying the veteran to a veteran's facility.

The family caregiver who is the primary provider of personal care services will receive in addition:

- Mental health services
- Respite care of not less than 30 days
- Medical care
- A monthly stipend.

The law authorizes the following related to mental healthcare:

- Readjustment counseling and related mental health services
- Prohibition of copayments from veterans who are catastrophically disabled
- An increase in dollars to disabled veterans for improvements and structural alterations as part of home health services
- Other programs related to the coordination of care, educational initiatives and special studies such as suicide rates.

The law authorizes the following related to women veterans:

- A study of barriers for women to receive healthcare from the VA
- Training and certification for mental healthcare providers for veterans suffering from sexual trauma and PTSD
- Healthcare services to a newborn child of a woman veteran receiving maternity care at a veteran's facility
- Several other initiatives related to counseling and child care.

The law authorizes the following related to rural health improvements:

- A program to provide readjustment and mental healthcare services to veterans such as peer outreach and peer support
- Services to immediate family members to assist in the readjustment of the veteran (including the family) to civilian life
- Travel reimbursement for veteran to veteran's facilities
- Grants to veteran's service organizations for transportation of veterans in highly rural areas.

The law also establishes a nonprofit research corporation to provide a flexible funding mechanism to conduct research, education, or both at veteran's medical centers.

13.3 Family and Medical Leave Act of 1993 (FMLA) (P.L. 103–3)

This Act is a federal law requiring covered employers to provide employees job-protected and unpaid leave for qualified medical and family reasons including personal and family illness, family military leave, pregnancy, adoption, or foster care placement of a child. Eligible employees can take up to 12 work weeks of unpaid leave during any 12 month period for the serious health condition of the employee, parent, spouse, or child or for pregnancy or care of a newborn child, or for adoption or foster care of a child.

13.4 Lifespan Respite Care Act of 2006 (P.L. 109–442)

This Act awards matching grants or cooperative agreements to eligible state agencies to: (1) expand and enhance respite care services to family caregivers; (2) improve the statewide dissemination and coordination of respite care; and (3) provide, supplement, or improve access and quality of respite care services to family caregivers, thereby reducing family caregiver strain (Navaie Waliser et al. 2002).

Title VII of the Public Health Service Act (PHSA) the Geriatric Education Center (GEC) Program provides students with clinical training in geriatrics in nursing homes, chronic and acute disease hospitals, ambulatory care centers, and senior centers.

Medicaid Home and Community Based Waiver Programs under the Social Security Act provide community support services to Medicaid beneficiaries who would otherwise require institutional care, including respite care, home modifications and non-medical transportation.

Social Services Block Grant Program (SSBG) enables States to meet the needs of residents to achieve or maintain economic self-sufficiency to prevent, reduce or eliminate dependency on social services. SSBGs fund a variety of initiatives including daycare, services to persons with disabilities, transportation, home delivered meals and independent/transitional living.

White House Task Force on the Middle Class (2009)[5] was created by President Obama to ensure that the economic challenges facing the middle class remain front and center in the work of the Administration. This included attention to Balancing Work and Family Responsibilities, in particular supporting family caregivers. This Task Force worked with the Department of Health and Human Services to develop a New Caregiver Initiative in the Fiscal Year 2011 Budget that provides a total of $ 50 million in additional funds for the National Family Caregiver Support Program and the Native American Caregiver Support Program.

These programs provide temporary respite care, counseling and training and help with retrofitting homes to accommodate the needs of aging relatives. They also link caregivers with information and referrals to other supports. The extra funding will allow nearly 200,000 additional caregivers to be served and 3 million more hours of respite care to be provided.

The Caregiver initiative also adds $ 50 million in funding to programs that provide transportation assistance for medical and other appointments, adult day care, and in-home services such as aides to help seniors bathe, cook, and clean. This initiative is also focused on caregivers to the elderly. The Lifespan Respite Care Program, which will double in size, is designed to help families caring for people of all ages with disabilities.

The Task Force also studied the need for additional support for easing the financial burden of caregiving, especially recommending giving tax credits to primary caregivers of people with long-term care needs.

These various federal and State programs offer direct or indirect services which affect the pool of caregivers and the quality of caregiving. The scope of these programs is often limited; they may vary in organization, management and funding by State. Generally there is limited data on the effectiveness of these programs (O'Shaughnessy 2012). One of the built-in problems of federal and State caregiving initiatives is the uncertainty of funding from fiscal year to fiscal year. This uncertainty is a major distraction to maintaining the momentum and quality of programs and limits their effectiveness. Nonetheless, several States have managed to enact

[5] See the *Annual Report of the White House Task Force on the Middle Class*, November, 2010, Office of the Vice President, Chaired by Vice President Joe Biden. http://www.whitehouse.gov/sites/default/files/microsites/100226-annual-report-middle-class.pdf.

laws establishing paid family leave. Some States identify family caregivers during the process in which they apply for Medicaid and refer them to eligible caregiving services (Feinberg et al. 2011).[6]

13.5 New Models of Caregiving

The Institute of Medicine's (IOM) Committee on the Needs of the Future Healthcare Workforce identified three key principles that need to form the basis of a system of care delivery for older Americans. They are: (1) healthcare needs need to be addressed comprehensively; (2) provided efficiently; and (3) involve persons as active partners in their own care. The Committee reviewed numerous models of caregiving; many models were innovative but lacked rigorous evaluation, and therefore could not be replicated in other settings (Institute of Medicine 2008). However, there were several characteristics common to the new innovative vigorously evaluated programs of caregiving (Boult et al. 2007). The Committee concluded that a variety of models would need to be used to meet the targeted needs of older Americans because their health needs are so diverse. Similarly, caregiver support programs may not be sufficient for older adults with more intensive needs. Furthermore, the models may not produce the same results in all settings. Given these caveats the characteristics that appeared to be intrinsic to successful innovative programs were: interdisciplinary team care, case management, chronic disease self-management, pharmaceutical management, preventive home visits, proactive rehabilitation, caregiver education and support, and transitional care.

While the Affordable Care Act is still being tweaked as plans turn toward its full implementation, it has the potential of increasing access to primary care services, reducing administrative barriers, and facilitating coordination across the continuum of care for the delivery of high quality, patient-centered care (Davis et al. 2011). However, the Act should also embrace health promotion and disease prevention as these have a greater impact on health status than do healthcare services. Evidence indicates that preventive interventions targeting the root causes of disease account for about 80% of the reduction in morbidity and mortality we have achieved (Hardcastle et al. 2011).

Long-term care should envelope long-term well-being throughout all decades of life. Education about what we know best for maintaining people's health and well-being is essential in preventing or delaying the early onset of debilitating illnesses (Turiel 2005). As the Institute of Medicine Committee noted, the key components of caregiving for the elderly begin much earlier than the age of 65. Innovations in the healthcare of the elderly begin with incentives and support for healthy lifestyles before chronic disease limits patients' choices.

---

[6] See the Family Caregiver Alliance website for federal and state legislation and policy reports and initiatives that directly impact caregivers of older adults and adults with disabilities. http://caregiver.org/caregiver/jsp/content_node.jsp?nodeid=2324&chcategory=30.

13.6 Summary

As more of us gain additional years in longevity and the needs of our aging population become more diverse and complex, the number of family and other informal caregivers and their limited training, has become problematic. While historically the family was the major caregiver for its aging and sick members, providing care to members with functional limitations and chronic impairments has become emotionally and physically costly to carers especially in the case of severe dementias requiring full care. There is a need for a national comprehensive, coordinated plan for carers especially with the baby boomer generation reaching retirement age. As of 2011 and every day for the next 19 years, 10,000 baby boomers will reach 65 according to the Pew Foundation.

There are resources and initiatives currently available from national and State levels but most are inadequately funded, lack evaluation of their effectiveness, and are not well publicized. The recently passed Affordable Care Act is an attempt to provide greater access to primary care services, reduce barriers, and facilitate coordination across the continuum of care. The Act should also embrace health promotion and disease prevention as these have a greater impact on health status than do health services. The Act, ideally, should evaluate initiatives as they are implemented so that effectiveness and efficiency can be assessed.

13.7 Questions for Discussion

1. Have gains in the quantity of life outpaced quality in people's added years? Discuss.
2. What, in your opinion, should be some key guiding principles that underlie caregiving in our country?
3. Discuss the strengths and weaknesses of the Affordable Care Act.
4. What is meant by "long-term care"?
5. As the proportion of minority populations increases over time, especially those minorities with higher prevalence of certain chronic diseases, the growing diversity of the older population in the U.S. will influence the types of services expected and the rates of utilization. Discuss.

References

Berkman, L. F., & Glymour, M. M. (2006). How society shapes aging: The centrality of variability. *Daedalus, 135*(1), 105–114.

Boult, C., Green, A., Boult, L. B., Pascala, J. T., Snyder, C., & Left, B. (2007). *Successful models of comprehensive healthcare for multi-morbid older persons: A review of effects on health and healthcare.* Paper commissioned by the IOM committee on the future healthcare workforce for older Americans.

Davis, K., Abrams, M., & Stremikis, K. (2011). How the Affordable Care Act will strengthen the nation's primary care foundation. *Journal of General Internal Medicine, 26*(10), 1201–1203.
Elmore, D. L., & Talley, R. C. (2009). Family caregiving and U.S. federal policy. In S. H. Qualls & S. H. Zarit (Eds.), *Aging families and caregiving* (pp. 209–231). New York: Wiley.
Families USA (2011). The Affordable Care Act: Provisions that will help caregivers. Washington, DC. www.familiesusa.org. Accessed 10 February 2013.
Feinberg, L. F., & Newman, S. L. (2004). A study of 10 states since passage of the National Family Caregiver Support Program: Policies, perceptions, and program development. *The Gerontologist, 44*(6), 760–769.
Feinberg, L. F., Newman, S. L., Gray, L., Kolb, K. N., & Fox-Grage, W. (Nov 2004). *The state of the states in family caregiver support: A 50-state study*. National Center on Caregiving, National Caregiving Alliance and National conference of State Legislatures.
Feinberg, L. F., Reinhard, S. C., Houser, A., & Choula, R. (2011). *Valuing the invaluable: 2011 update. The growing contributions and costs of family caregiving*. AARP Public Policy Institute, Washington, DC. www.aarp.org/ppi. Accessed 11 February 2013.
Hacker, J. S. (Ed.). (2008). *Health at risk: America's ailing health system—and how to heal it*. New York: Columbia University Press.
Hardcastle, L. E., Record, K. L., Jacobson, P. D., & Gostin, L. O. (2011). Improving the population's health: The Affordable Care Act and the importance of integration. *Journal of Law, Medicine & Ethics, 39*(3), 317–327.
Hudson, R. B. (2011). *America's opportunity: The potential of an aging society*. Public policy and aging report. National academy on an aging society. A policy institute of the Gerontological Society of America (Vol. 21, No. 4). Fall, Washington, DC.
Institute of Medicine. (2008). *Retooling for an aging America: Building the healthcare workforce*. Washington, DC: The National Academies Press.
Kaiser Family Foundation (2010). *Focus on health reform. Summary of new health reform law. Patient protection and affordable care act* (P.L. 111–148). http://www.kff.org/healthreform/upload/8061.pdf. Accessed 25 February 2010.
Kelly, K. (28 Sep 2010). *Supporting caregivers across the lifespan: Federal initiatives and technical assistance for program development*. 2010 National Home & Community-based services conference. Family Caregiving Alliance, National Center on Caregiving, San Francisco, CA.
McGlynn, E. A., Meltzer, D., & Hacker, J. S. (2008). Just how good is American medical care? In J. S. Hacker (Ed.), *Health at risk. America's ailing health system—and how to heal it* (pp. 88–105). New York: Columbia University Press.
Mechanic, D. (2006). *The truth about healthcare: Why reform is not working in America* (pp. 51–66). New Brunswick: Rutgers University Press.
Mechanic, D. (2012). Seizing opportunities under the Affordable Care Act for transforming the mental and behavioral health system. *Health Affairs, 31*(2), 376–382.
Metlife Mature Market Institute (2008). *The Metlife study of caregiving costs to working caregivers: Double jeopardy for baby boomers caring for their parents*. Mature Market Institute @ metlife.com.
Mintz, S., Feinberg, L. F., Horvath, J., Hunt, G., Plooster, L., Kagin, J., Levine, C., Lynn, J., & Wilkinson, A. (2003). *Family caregiving and public policy principles for change*. www.caregiver.com/articles/general/.family_caregiving_public_policy. htm. Accessed 1 March 2012.
Navaie Waliser, M., Feldman, P. H., Gould, D. A., Levine, C., Kuerbis, A. N., & Donelan, K. (2002). When the caregiver needs care: The plight of vulnerable caregivers. *American Journal of Public Health, 92*(3), 409–413.
O'Shaughnessy, C. V. (20 July 2012). *Family caregivers: The primary providers of assistance to people with functional limitations and chronic impairments*. Background paper No. 84, National Health Policy Forum. The George Washington University, Washington, DC. www.nhpf@gwu.org. Accessed 1 March 2012.

Rowe, J. W. (2011). Successful societal adaptation to the aging of America. In R. B. Hudson (Ed.), *America's opportunity: The potential of an aging society* (pp. 11–16). Public policy and aging report. Washington, DC: National Academy on an Aging Society.
Rowe, J. W., & Kahn, R. I. (1998). *Successful aging*. New York: Dell.
Stone, R. I. (2000). *Long-term care for the elderly with disabilities: Current policy, emerging trends, and implications for the twenty-first century*. Milbank Memorial fund, New York.
Turiel, J. S. (2005). *Our parents ourselves. How American healthcare imperils middle age and beyond*. Berkeley: University of California Press.

[illegible]

Chapter 14
Caregivers' Utilization of Social Networks and Social Media

14.1 Introduction

Maintaining relationships with others is often difficult for caregivers (George and Gwyther 1986; Pillemer and Suitor 1996). A common finding is that an individual's involvement with family and friends declines after they become a primary caregiver, especially a caregiver to a person with dementia.[1] The demands of dementia caregiving are generally higher than those of nondementia caregiving, and the duration is longer (Ory et al. 1999). Therefore, the degree of stress will vary with the caregiver's appraisal of the situation (Lawton et al. 1991), including the variability in the progression of symptoms, difficult and unsafe behaviors, and ability to sustain personal care (Neufeld and Kushner 2009).

As a result of technological advances and social trends, people are taking advantage of new opportunities to experience the healing power of affirming human connections on the Internet (Langshur 2008). Caregivers increasingly are using online social tools to gather information, share experiences, and discuss concerns (Fox 2011). People caring for loved ones are more likely than other adults to use social network sites to gather and share health information and support.

The role of caregiver differs in relation to the health conditions and disabilities of the care receiver and variations in the level of intensity and frequency of caregiving activities. In general, time is limited for face-to-face interaction with others because caregivers are running errands, keeping doctor's appointments, and meeting the daily needs of sick and elderly loved ones. The feelings of obligation and the associated guilt of not being present when needed frequently causes caregivers to restrict their social networks.[2] On the other hand, depending on the care recipient's physical and mental condition and need for constant vigilance, the caregiver may be able to join a self-help group in real or virtual time and use respite services

[1] Caregiving can also have a serious impact on the relationship with the caregiver's spouse (Kleban et al. 1989).

[2] With respect to caregiving to dementia patients, the shame associated with mental illness may cause some caregivers to isolate themselves and rely on resources within the household. See Bickel and Jones (1989).

J. G. Bruhn, H. M. Rebach, *The Sociology of Caregiving*,
Clinical Sociology: Research and Practice, DOI 10.1007/978-94-017-8857-1_14,

Table 14.1 Reasons online health information seekers used the internet to connect with others. (Source: JupiterResearch. Online Health: Assessing the risks and opportunity of social and one-to-one media, 2007)

	% of seekers
To see what other consumers say about a medication or treatment	36
To research other consumers' knowledge and experiences	31
To learn skills or get education that helps me manage a condition	27
To get emotional support	17
To build awareness around a disease or cause	15
To share my knowledge of and experiences with a medication or treatment	14
To share my knowledge of and experience with a health issue	14
To find consumers' recommendations and opinions about hospitals and other treatment options	13
To find consumers' recommendations and opinions about hospitals and other treatment centers	13
To find consumers' recommendations and opinions about doctors	10
To feel I belong to a group or community	8
None of the above	22

to maintain their more important social networks (Wright 2000; Russell 2004). A strong cyber-support system can help when the caregiver is dealing with powerful emotions, yet wants to retain their anonymity (Colvin et al. 2004). Social media is appealing to many caregivers because it widens their universe of information and opinion, and shares interests and concerns. (See Table 14.1). Connecting with other caregivers can foster hope, provide information and guidance, and share emotional support (Sarasohn-Kahn 2008).

14.1.1 Definitions

Social networks are broadly defined here as a set of contacts by which an individual keeps their social identity, receives emotional support, practical assistance, services, information, and the ability to develop meaningful relationships (Bordogna and Olivadeti 2012). Social networks have considerable influence on individual health; they can act as buffers for high levels of stress and protect against early mortality.

Social media is defined as forms of electronic communication through which users create online communities to share information, ideas, personal messages, and other content with other stakeholders. Different types of social media include collaborative projects such as Wikipedia, blogs, social networking sites such as Facebook, Twitter, and MySpace, content communities such as YouTube, and virtual worlds like Second Life. Online support groups, forums, podcasts, wikis, discussion groups and communities are also included under "social media" (Graab 2012). Social media's major assets are showing caregivers that they are not alone and they can be themselves (Buckwalter and Davis 2002).

Social support is defined here as giving and receiving tangible or emotional assistance, empathy, validation, or information (Vaux 1998). The buffering model suggests that social support buffers the deleterious effects of stress over time (Rook 1990).

The objectives of this chapter are to discuss the advantages and disadvantages of social networks and social media as sources of social support for caregivers and their use of these resources.

14.1.2 Scope of Internet Use

According to a survey conducted by the Pew Foundation during 2009–2010, 30 % of adults in the U.S. perform the functions of a caregiver in some way. Eight in ten of these caregivers have some access to the Internet. Of these, 88 % look online for health information ranging from certain treatments to hospital ratings to end-of-life decisions. Being a caregiver in and of itself is associated with a greater likelihood of using the internet, especially to access health information (Pew Internet Project 2012). Caregivers in the Pew survey were active healthcare consumers and highly social both online and offline. For example, currently, there are more that 50 million American boomers on Facebook, many of whom are active caregivers.

The age group 18–33 is still the largest user of social media (Chou et al. 2009). Adults 45 and older doubled their social networking use in the period between 2008 and 2010. Adults 74 years and older have quadrupled their social networking participation. Baby Boomers who are caring for their aging parents are heavier social media users than their non-caregiving counterparts.[3]

[3] Two recent studies examined the role of technology and family caregiving. "Home Tweet Home: The Age Lesson Boomer Media Study" used a panel of baby boomer caregivers to determine how they used their time on the web. The caregivers were using the web to find health information and community resources. They also use a variety of sites to manage finances, coordinate care, make appointments, and arrange support services and monitor medications for their parents and other relatives. The top site for these baby boomer caregivers is Facebook. See http://www.agelessons.com/joomla21.

United Healthcare and the National Alliance for Caregiving conducted a study "e-Connected Family Caregivers: Bringing Caregiving into the 21st Century" in November, 2010. They surveyed 1,000 family caregivers. Caregivers had the greatest receptivity to personal health records, caregiving coordination systems, caregiver training simulations, and caregiving decision support systems. Caregivers under age 50 were the most receptive to new technologies. Of those surveyed, 70 % said that they had used the internet for caregiving related information or support. The most trusted sources of information were medical websites such as WebMD, the Mayo Clinic.com or government websites like Medicare or Administration on Aging, or consumer review websites. See http://www.caregiving.org/data/Fact_Sheet_e-Connected_Family_Caregiver_study.pdf.

14.2 The Support Role of Social Networks and Social Media

Caregiving is basically a solitary activity carried out in caregiver-care receiver dyads. Taking on the role of caregiver usually involves significant changes in social networks for the caregiver and care receiver. Frequently the social networks of care receivers shrink for reasons of age, health, relocation, or neglect and non-use, while the social networks of caregivers require re-alignment, reconfiguration, limitations and new connections. It is widely accepted that as needs and resources change with age, individual's social networks undergo transformations. Face-to-face interactions may be replaced by virtual connections or other compensatory processes. Rook and Schuster (1996) have called this "relationship specialization" or the idea that different networks provide different kinds of social support.[4] Older adults expand or realign their social networks in response to network disruptions and losses. Social media may be the means by which some caregivers maintain connectedness to others and reduce their own vulnerability to adverse mental and physical health outcomes.

Few studies have focused specifically on caregivers' use of online social support. One study by Bass et al. (1998) investigated whether ComputerLink, a computer support intervention for family caregivers of homebound individuals with complex disorders such as Alzheimer patients, reduced their levels of care-related strain. After 1 year the experimental group showed a reduction in certain types of strain for caregivers who were spouses, who had larger informal support networks, or who did not live with their care receivers. For nonspousal caregivers who were initially more stressed or who lived with a care receiver, the frequent use of ComputerLink was associated with more strain.

Several potential benefits of online social support for caregivers include enabling caregivers to use the Internet at a time, place and pace convenient for them; anonymity can facilitate caregivers asking sensitive questions; computer mediated communication has the potential for meeting individual caregiver needs; and a computer based intervention could increase the options for delivering services to caregivers of Alzheimer's patients.

Colvin et al. (2004) obtained the cooperation of 15 Websites in the U.S. and Canada offering caregiver online networks to recruit the participation of 77 caregivers who responded to questions concerning their perceptions of online social support. About half of the respondents were caring for persons with Alzheimer's disease. Respondents' caregiving involved them for an average of 6.8 h per week.

The advantages of computer-mediated communication (CMC) were identified as anonymity, asynchrony, and connectivity or the ability to personalize use of CMC. The advantage of anonymity made it easier to relate and fostered a nonjudgmental atmosphere online. With less judgment there was a willingness to bond and help one another. The convenience and suitability of an online group and the immediacy of information and response to questions made the availability of social support

[4] See the use of telephone support groups. Bank et al. (2006). Also, Goodman and Pynoos (1988).

synchronous with the caregivers' schedule. There was always someone online. CMC was personalized to meet the needs of caregivers.

A major advantage of CMC was the ability to find and expand the network of status-similar others who were willing to share information and solutions to problems. Several caregivers who used CMC indicated that connecting with others gave them understanding and acceptance of the shortcomings of caregiving.

Online groups have disadvantages, too. Although computer-mediated communication is cost effective, caregivers must have access to a computer and to the Internet. Lack of visual, aural, and contextual cues contribute to the relative impersonal nature of online communication. Since health professionals do not facilitate most publically accessible online groups, opportunities for inaccuracies and mistaken medical information is always present. Online relationships should supplement, not replace, real life social interactions (White and Dorman 2001).

14.3 Network Disruptions: A Predictor of Caregiver Distress

Interestingly, several studies of Alzheimer caregivers found that negative interactions were particularly predictive of caregiver distress. Fiore et al. (1983) and his associates studied both supportive and upsetting aspects of spousal Alzheimer's caregivers social networks. They found that experiencing upset within the network due to unmet expectations or to negative interactions with others was the best predictor of caregiver depression (Neufeld and Kushner 2009).

Semple's (1992) study of family conflict in Alzheimer's caregiving families also provides support of interpersonal stress as a predictor of psychological stress. In a study of 555 caregivers, conflict over family members' attitudes and actions toward the caregiver were related to depression. The factors included were: not telephoning enough, not giving the caregiver enough help, not showing enough appreciation for one's work as a caregiver, and giving the caregiver unwanted advice. Other studies of stressful aspects of roles, e.g. mother, wife, have found interpersonal stress with intimates appears to be a powerful predictor of caregiver distress. This finding, along with reports that a caregiver's involvement with family and friends declines after they become a caregiver, sets the stage for caregiver burden.

Birkel and Jones (1989) found, in addition, that the presence of dementia can actually *decrease* the amount of help others provide to the care recipient. Families of dementia patients rely on resources within their household and therefore are less likely to receive help from persons outside the household. Indeed, this study indicates that responsibility for caring for nondemented individuals is shared to a greater extent than the care of demented persons. Becoming an Alzheimer's caregiver appears to reduce social interaction and increases the risk of caregiver burden (Prince and Bell-Scott 1996).

Caregiving has both positive and negative effects on family caregivers.[5] Caregiving is demanding and stressful, but it can also be a source of positive feelings such as feeling good, confident and satisfied about oneself (Hwang et al. 2011). Caregivers with low social support and a low sense of control perceive the caregiver role as more burdensome. Also caring for persons with severe comorbid conditions can decrease a caregiver's sense of control. Perceived availability of social support appears to moderate the negative effects of caregiving (Neufeld and Harrison 2010). However, the presence of support does not make caregiving for a family member with dementia easier (Wuest and Stern 2001).[6]

Caregivers play a large role in socialization and communication for the people they care for. Empathic listening, using appropriate language, and understanding how perceptions and nonverbal expressions can cause positive or negative reactions by care recipients is critical in caregiving.

14.4 Telephone Networks

The telephone network is a new concept in social support to caregivers (Goodman and Pynoos 1988). The Telephone Support Group (TSG) project began in 2002 as a federally funded program. Goals of the project included reaching isolated family caregivers not being served by in-person groups. When support groups are offered over the telephone many caregivers are able to participate who are otherwise unable to attend in person groups. Offering groups over the telephone via conference call eliminates or reduces many of the barriers to traditional support group participation including physical limitations of the caregiver, the discomfort in a group setting, distance, transportation, or inability to leave a care recipient alone at home (Smith and Toseland 2006). Bank et al. (2006) found telephone-based support groups useful among White American and Cuban American dementia caregivers in the Miami area. Support groups were conducted over the telephone in English and in Spanish. Eighty-one percent of the participants found the groups valuable because of the social and emotional support and information obtained from other group members. Bank concluded that telecommunications technology can overcome logistical barriers to joining a support group and can provide benefits similar to those obtained in face-to-face groups. Eisdorfer et al. (2003) found that technology-based interventions resulted in a decrease in caregiver depression and caregiver stress.

[5] See the use of telephone support groups. Bank et al. (2006). Also, Goodman and Pynoos (1988).

[6] Negative reactions by care recipients to their being helped is a possible source of caregiver distress. Recent studies indicate that many care recipients experience some negative reactions to assistance with daily activities. Reports indicate that one third to two thirds of recipients report some negative reactions to help, and a number of studies have shown that negative reactions are associated with depression or other measures of psychological distress (Newsom 1999). Some care recipients have reported lowered self-esteem in response to help, feelings of rejection, dependency, anger, resentment, concerns about reciprocity, and feelings of incompetence. Negative reactions ranged from receiving either too little or too much help.

14.5 Interventions to Moderate Family Caregiver Burden and Stress

Caregiver and family needs vary across the course of a disease as well as in response to life changes. Information and services available at one point in time may not be helpful at another, therefore, periodic assessment of needs is necessary. The advantage of social networks and social media is that they are available to caregivers in a variety of forms at times they are needed. Toseland et al. (1990) found that an individual intervention such as counseling had more positive effects on caregiver psychological functioning and well-being than did a group intervention, whereas a group intervention produced greater improvements in coping with caregiver stress. Therefore, the most appropriate type of intervention is best determined by the types of problems and issues specific to an individual caregiver.

Support groups are the most popular interventions available to caregivers. Studies have shown that participants in support groups evaluate these as useful and helpful (Toseland et al. 1990). In addition, there is some evidence that they provide knowledge and enhance informal support networks (Bourgeois et al. 1996). Programs which offer a combination of counseling, education and support have been found to be especially effective (Mittelman et al. 1996).

Multi-component programs have been found to meet the needs of individual caregivers and to have positive effects on caregivers in subjective burden caregiver depression, stress levels, service utilization, and perceived quality of life (Mittleman et al. 1996; Zarit et al. 1998). There is some evidence that culturally-targeted education and training interventions can be more effective with Latinas and Caucasian women than a traditional support group in reducing caregiver depression, increasing positive coping and fostering social support (Gallagher-Thompson et al. 2000, 2001). These findings suggest further research with interventions among ethnic minority caregivers is needed. Galanti (2008) has provided a comprehensive and sensitive guidebook of information to help in caring for persons from a variety of ethnic groups. Cultural competence can often reduce stress in caregiving and lead to better outcomes for the caregiver and receiver.

There needs to be more research on how technological advances can improve caregiver outcomes. Home videos, telephone services, computer programs, online education and support are such examples (Coon et al. 1999). There is little evidence that interventions aimed at supporting and/or providing information to carers of people with dementia are uniformly effective (Thompson et al. 2007). While caregiver burden can be reduced to some degree, it is rarely possible to eliminate it completely (Sorensen et al. 2002).

14.6 Summary

Caregiving can be physically and emotionally isolating and isolation, in turn, can create an environment that can lead to carer burnout, especially as the care recipient's condition deteriorates and there is a need for a continual caregiver presence.

While no set of interventions can completely resolve the stresses of caregiving, there are ways to minimize caregiver's burdens. Social networks and social media are ways caregivers can retain connections with friends and family and develop new links with other caregivers. These linkages can be informational, educational and supportive and used as the needs of caregivers change. This has been referred to as "relationship specialization." Different networks and media provide different kinds of support.

Computer-mediated communication (CMC) has been used to offer online networks and personalize them to meet the needs of caregivers. Telephone support groups have reduced many of the barriers to participation in traditional support groups. Such technology-based interventions have resulted in a decrease in caregiver's stress and depression. Programs which offer a combination of counseling, education and support have been found to be especially effective for caregivers. It is important to develop culturally-targeted interventions to meet the needs of caregivers from different ethnic and racial groups.

14.7 Questions for Discussion

1. Discuss in what ways a cyber-support system can be supportive to caregivers.
2. What are some of the disadvantages of a caregiver becoming involved in social networks?
3. What are some reasons for inconsistencies in the effectiveness of interventions with caregivers?
4. What are some methodological issues in studying intervention effectiveness?
5. Discuss why young caregivers may experience increased caregiver burden.

References

Bank, A. L., Arguelles, S., Rubert, M., Eisdorfer, C., & Czaja, S. J. (2006). The value of telephone support groups among ethnically diverse caregivers of persons with dementia. *Gerontologist, 46*(1), 134–138.

Bass, D. M., McClendon, M. J., Brennan, P. F., & McCarthy, C. (1998). The buffering effect of a computer support network on caregiver strain. *Journal of Aging & Health, 10*(1), 20–43.

Birkel, R. C., & Jones, C. J. (1989). A comparison of the caregiving networks of dependent elderly individuals who are lucid and those who are demented. *Gerontologist, 29,* 114–119.

Bordogna, M. T., & Olivadoti, S. (2012). The role of social networks in health. *Sociology Study, 2*(1), 60–67.

Bourgeois, M., Schulz, R., & Burgio, L. (1996). Interventions for caregivers of patients with Alzheimer's disease: A review and analysis of content, process, and outcomes. *International Journal on Aging and Human Development, 43,* 35–92.

Brodaty, H., & Donkin, M. (2009). Family caregivers of people with dementia. *Dialogues in Clinical Neuroscience, 11*(2), 217–228.

Buckwalter, K. C., & Davis, L. L. (2002). Elder caregiving in rural communities. White paper commissioned by U.S. Dept. of Agriculture, Spring 2002, last updated 10/20/2010.

Chou, W. Y., Hunt, Y. M., Beckjord, E. B., Moser, R. P., & Hesse, B. W. (2009). Social media use in the United States: Implications for health communication. *Journal of Medical Internet Research, 11*(4), e48.

Colvin, J., Chenoweth, L., Bold, M., & Harding, C. (2004). Caregivers of older adults: Advantages and disadvantages of Internet-based social support. *Family Relations, 53*(1), 49–60.

Coon, D., Schulz, R., & Ory, M. (1999). Innovative intervention approaches with Alzheimer's disease caregivers. In D. Biegel & A. Blum (Eds.), *Innovations in practice and service delivery across the lifespan* (pp. 295–325). New York: Oxford University Press.

Eisendorfer, C., Czaja, S., Lowenstein, D., Rubert, M. P., Arguelles, S., Mitrani, V. B., & Szapocznik, J. (2003). The effect of a family therapy and technology-based intervention on caregiver depression. *Gerontologist, 43*(4), 521–531.

Fiore, J., Becker, J., & Coppel, D. B. (1983). Social network interactions: A buffer or a stress? *American Journal of Community Psychology, 11,* 423–439.

Fox, S. (2011). *The social life of health information.* Pew Research Center's Internet & American Life Project: Washington, DC. http://pewinternet.org/Reports/2011/Social-Life-of-health-info.aspx. Accessed 16 June 2013.

Galanti, G. (2008). *Caring for patients from different cultures* (4th Ed.). Philadelphia: University of Pennsylvania Press.

Gallagher-Thompson, D., Lovett, S., Rose, J., McKibbin, C., Coon, D., Futterman, A., & Thompson, L. (2000). Impact of psychoeducational interventions on distressed family caregivers. *Journal of Clinical Geropsychology, 6,* 91–110.

Gallagher-Thompson, D., Arean, P., Rivera, P., & Thompson, L. (2001). Reducing distress in Hispanic family caregivers using a psychoeducational intervention. *Clinical Gerontologist, 23,* 17–32.

George, L. K., & Gwyther, L. P. (1986). Caregiver well-being: A multidimensional examination of family caregivers of demented adults. *Gerontologist, 26,* 253–259.

Goodman, C. C., & Pynoos, J. (1988). Telephone networks connect caregiving families of Alzheimer's victims. *Gerontologist, 28*(5), 602–606.

Graab, D. (2012). Reaching caregivers via social media. Presentation at CMC Caregiving Coalition Conference. http://www.caring.com. Accessed 26 January 2012.

Hwang, B., Fleischmann, K. E., Howie-Esquivel, J., Stotts, N. A., & Dracup, K. (2011). Caregiving for patients with heart failure: Impact on patients' families. *American Journal of Critical Care, 20*(6), 431–441.

Kleban, M. H., Brody, E. M., Schoonover, C. B., & Hoffman, C. (1989). Family help to the elderly: Perceptions of sons-in-law regarding parent care. *Journal of Marriage and the Family, 51,* 303–312.

Langshur, S. (2008). *Online healthcare gets personal.* Chicago: CarePages, Inc.

Lawton, M. P., Moss, M., Kleban, M. H., Glicksman, A., & Rovine, M. (1991). A two-factor model of caregiving appraisal and psychological well-being. *Journals of Gerontology, 46,* P181–P189.

Mittelman, M., Ferris, S., Shulman, E., Steinberg, G., & Levin, B. (1996). Family intervention to delay nursing home placement of patients with Alzheimer's disease. *Journal of the American Medical Association, 276,* 1725–1731.

Neufeld, A., & Harrison, M. (2010). *Nursing and family caregiving: Social support and nonsupport.* New York: Springer.

Neufeld, A., & Kushner, K. E. (2009). Men family caregivers' experience of nonsupportive interactions. *Journal of Family Nursing, 15*(2), 171–191.

Newsome J. T. (1999). Another side to caregiving: Negative reactions to being helped. *Current Directions in Psychological Science, 8,* 183–187.

Ory, M. G., Hoffman, R. R., Yee, J. L., Tennstedt, S., & Schulz, R. (1999). Prevalence and impact of caregiving: A detailed comparison between dementia and nondementia caregivers. *The Gerontologist, 39,* 177–185.

Pew Internet and American Life Project. (2012). Family caregivers online, summary of findings. http://pewinternet.org/Reports/2012/Caregivers-online/Summary-of-Findings.aspx. Accessed 8 August 2012.

Pillemer, K., & Suitor, J. (1996). Family stress and social support among caregivers to persons with Alzheimer's disease. In G. R. Pierce, B. R. Sarason, & I. G. Sarason (Eds.), *Handbook of social support and the family* (pp. 467–494). New York: Plenum Press.

Price, C. A., & Bell-Scott (1996). Alzheimer's caregivers: Enhancing support group effectiveness. *Family Service Review, 9*(3/4), 231–245.

Rook, K. S. (1990). Stressful aspects of older adults' social relationships: Current theory and research. In M. A. Stephens, J. H. Crowther, S. E. Hobfoll, & D. L. Tennenbaum (Eds.), *Stress and coping in later-life families* (pp. 173–192). New York: Hemisphere.

Rook, K. S., & Schuster, T. L. (1996). Compensatory processes in the social networks of older adults. In G. R. Pierce, B. R. Sarason, & I. G. Sarason (Eds.), *Handbook of social support and the family* (pp. 219–248). New York: Plenum Press.

Russell, R. (2004). Social networks among elderly men caregivers. *The Journal of Men's Studies, 13*(1), 121–142.

Sarasohn-Kahn, J. (2008). *The wisdom of patients: Health care meets online social media.* Oakland: California Healthcare Foundation.

Semple, S. J. (1992). Conflict in Alzheimer caregiving families: Its dimensions and consequences. *Gerontologist, 32,* 648–655.

Smith, T., & Toseland, R. (2006). The effectiveness of a telephone support program for caregivers of frail older adults. *Gerontologist, 46*(5), 620–629.

Sorensen, S., Pinquart, M., & Duberstein, P. (2002). How effective are interventions with caregivers? An updated meta-analysis. *Gerontologist, 42*(3), 356–372.

Thompson, C. A., Spilsbury, K., Hall, J., Birks, Y., Barnes, C., & Adamson, J. (2007). Systematic review of information and support interventions for caregivers of people with dementia. *BMC Geriatrics, 7,* 18. Doi: 1186/1471-2318-7-18.

Toseland, R. W., Rossiter, C. M., Peak, T., & Smith, G. C. (1990). Comparative effectiveness of individual and group interventions to support family caregivers. *Social Work, 35*(3), 209–217.

Vaux, A. (1988). *Social support: Theory, research, and intervention.* New York: Praeger.

White, M., & Dorman, S. M. (2001). Receiving social support online: Implications for health education. *Health Education Research, 16*(6), 693–707.

Wright, K. (2000). Computer-mediated social support, older adults, and coping. *Journal of Communication, 50*(3), 100–118.

Wuest, J., Ericson, P. K., Stern, P. N., & Irwin, G. W. (2001). Connected and disconnected support: The impact on the caregiving process in Alzheimer's disease. *Health Care for Women International, 22,* 115–130.

Zarit, S., Stephens, M., Townsend, A., & Greene, R. (1998). Stress reduction for family caregivers: Effects of adult day care use. *Journal of Gerontology: Social Sciences, 53B,* S267–S277.

Index

J. G. Bruhn, H. M. Rebach, *The Sociology of Caregiving*,
Clinical Sociology: Research and Practice, DOI 10.1007/978-94-017-8857-1,

The manufacturer's authorised representative in the EU is Springer Nature Customer Service Centre GmbH, Europaplatz 3, 69115 Heidelberg, Germany. If you have any concerns regarding our products, please contact ProductSafety@springernature.com

Printed and bound by CPI Group (UK) Ltd, Croydon, CR0 4YY
30/09/2026
02225497-0007